W9-AMI-327

NO MORE
COLD HANDS, COLD FEET

**Out of the Deep Freeze: The Essential Guide to
Thyroid Problems**

**Do you suffer from hypothyroidism, thyroid
fatigue, a thyroid problem, cold hands and feet,
thyroid nodules, hair loss, dry skin, thyroid
storm, thyroiditis, thyroidectomy, thyroid
hormone, and thyroid medication questions?**

**All explained here in this entertaining book by a
#1 best selling medical author. Look no further
and figure out as Dr. Purser dives deeper!**

by Dan Purser MD
www.drpursernaturaloptions.com

COPYRIGHT STATEMENT for books

Copyright © 2015 by Dan Purser MD. All Rights Reserved.

No part of this publication may be reproduced, distributed, or transmitted in any form or by any means, including photocopying, recording, or other electronic or mechanical methods, or by any information storage and retrieval system without the prior written permission of the publisher, except in the case of very brief quotations embodied in critical reviews and certain other noncommercial uses permitted by copyright law.

Get the more Kindle health series books here: GreatMedEbooks.com Published by DP Publishing LLC.

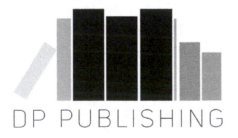

DP PUBLISHING

My Legal Protection

Do not use the information contained in this book to treat yourself. And this book is not meant to be the most thorough treatment on thyroid problems – it's written more for patients who cannot get to the bottom of their common problems (and questions) on thyroid issues and tribulations. Please consult with a knowledgeable physician in your area before starting or changing any treatment as might possibly be suggested in this book. I will not be held responsible if something goes wrong. So BE CAREFUL!

Thank you.

Dan Purser MD

FOREWORD

Women and men come into my office all the time with fatigue, cold hands and feet, dry skin and constipation all the time. They've begged their doctors to look at thyroid problems. Sometimes their doctor puts them on a "little L-thyroxine" and I'm never sure if this is just to mollify the patient or to assuage their own guilt in not really knowing what to do – but it makes me sad.

My incredibly hard working and overworked "brothers" and "sisters" in the medical field are doing all they can do – they are immensely overwhelmed and feel horribly underpaid. And now there is so much misinformation and "old physician's wives tales" out there that I feel the need to put this out for consideration.

I had the luck and opportunity to get to do research and work with one of the top pituitary endocrinologists on the west coast and I took a LOT of notes. Here it is – distilled and referenced for you and your physician to consider.

This is in the new "story approach" (for me at least) or better yet "allegorical approach" that has been used for generations to teach (as those who know will recognize it from the Bible or Koran) so I hope it makes it more interesting – my readers seem to like it immensely.

Good luck. And thanks for reading.

Dan Purser MD

Want to Connect with Dr. Purser?

For women's information on progesterone, testosterone and more download some awesome FREE reports:

www.drpursergifts4women.com

© Copyright by Dan Purser MD of Medutainment, Inc.

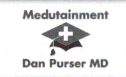

Sign up TODAY to Get Your FREE Reports!

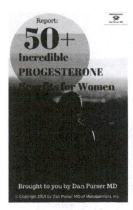
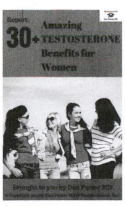
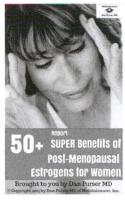

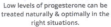

Low levels of progesterone can be treated naturally & optimally in the right situations.	An AMAZING LIST every woman should own -- all REFERENCED! NO FOOLING.	Learn the SUPER BENEFITS of Estrogens in Post-Menopausal Women! This report is fully referenced just for you!

Table of Contents

Chapter 1 – Thyroid is a Great Hormone
..................**Page 10**

Chapter 2 – True Facts and More Benefits of Thyroid
..................**Page 19**

Chapter 3 – Monitoring and Checking Levels
..................**Page 38**

Chapter 4 – Thyroid Practice Gems
..................**Page 41**

Chapter 5 – Why is Free T4 Important?
..................**Page 43**

Chapter 6 – Vitamins and Minerals for Thyroid Function
..................**Page 44**

Chapter 7 – Essential Oils That Support Thyroid Function
..................Page 54

Chapter 8 – Hashimoto's Thyroiditis
..................**Page 57**

Chapter 9 – Grave's Disease
..................**Page 63**

Chapter 10 – Reverse T3 – What it Means
..................**Page 64**

Chapter 11 – Side Effects and Problems
..................**Page 71**

Index
..................**Page 77**

Her Hair Was Scraggly...

Her chart said she was 32, *if* I'd done the math right (always questionable on a Monday morning).

But she looked (and acted) like she felt older. She moved slowly, deliberately – as if through a fog, as we talked. She'd come from Hawaii to see me – I felt honored like I always do. And humbled.

"I'm tired all the time. Exhausted. Plus hair loss – comes out in clumps after I shower. And weight gain I can't lose," She looked at me. "No matter what I do."

"Cold hands and feet?" I reached out to take her hand.

She hesitated then put her hand in mine as if to shake it weakly. She was immaculately dressed. It was apparent she came from money. But her hand was ice cold. And very dry.

I looked at her. "Your hand is freezing! Is this why you live in Hawaii?"

She gave a little laugh. "My husband's older, and very successful. I told him I was cold all the time and loved it there so we moved. He can run his business from home. We're from Vancouver...mostly..."

I nodded. "Constipated?"

"Yes," she said, a question on her face, wondering how I knew. "I have to take stool softeners all the time. People think I'm anorexic or something."

"Sick a lot?"

She nodded. "More than I should be…"

"How'd you hear about me?"

"My friend Courtney said you'd figure it out or die trying. I've been to like ten different doctors over there and in Canada – always the same -- non-answer answers." She looked at me – squarely in the face, questioning. "Or they say they just don't know."

"Check your thyroid?

"Yes, a TSH." She slid some papers forward. "Always the same – say it's normal. But I tell them it's my thyroid."
"One doctor put me on some, because I nagged him. And begged." She looked up at me. "But it only made me feel worse."

Half measures, I thought, but said, "Feels like your thyroid – your hands are ice cold, *and very dry*. Hair loss. Fatigue. Constipation."

I tapped the table with my pen, on her chart – I didn't use an EMR – didn't take insurance so no need too. Plus it made things too impersonal. And it's not private enough for my high-end patients. "Gonna be here a while?"

"I'm staying up at Sundance for the week. Or as long as it takes…"

"Seen Bob Redford?"

She laughed a little and shook her head. "No."

"Can we draw some blood? Do some tests?"

She studied my face. "Same ol' same ol'?"

I reassured. "No, we're going to dive deeper and figure this out. If you don't mind."

She teared up. Just a little. Caught me by surprise. She'd been disappointed but was on a journey. She was determined. I liked it – she was spunky. Despite being cold here in Utah, she was ready to face her problems. She very quietly said, "No, I don't mind. It's why I'm here."

I got up. "Come with me…"

(To Be Continued)

CHAPTER 1

THYROID IS A GREAT HORMONE

Thyroid IS a great hormone – easy to take with levels that are easy to follow but conversely thyroid hormone supplementation can be controversial and seemingly complicated.

I am NOT set in my ways on this and will use L-thyroxine (yes, the HORROR – I do use Synthroid® on occasion), or desiccated animal thyroid (such as ® or NatureThroid®) according to which I feel is best for the patient or situation (yes, I must make the referring doctor happy too). I'll also use Levothroid® and Cytomel® and others – there are many different names and brands. And different patients may sometimes need different brands[1].

Clearly, we have known for many decades that the majority of patients benefit from T4 and T3[2] (for a number of reasons supported by many studies[3] and hard opinions[4] which we detail[5]). Armour® Thyroid is a proven quality product and it contains T4, T3, T2, and T1 and treated levels rise in a clearly controlled and proper manner reflective of appropriate dosing (while the FDA has repeatedly found Synthroid® and the research behind it to be problematic leading to millions of dollars in fines and class action lawsuits[6]). We also believe that measuring and following TSH levels alone are not that helpful and it's clearly best to also follow Free T3 levels[7], since this is the active thyroid hormone at the cellular level, and to optimize those levels as done repeatedly throughout major studies[8] (or you won't get the same results).

My Personal Beliefs on Thyroid Dosing and Manner

Start with 1 grain (60 mg) a day. For older people start with ¼ or ½ grain a day

Increase at no more than 1 grain per month. Take in the morning (if your patient is taking once per day) on an empty stomach 30 minutes before eating for an optimal result – but always take on an empty stomach[9].

Optimized Levels

Supported in numerous studies (conflicted in others) your Free T3 level should be 3.9 pg/ml or above (up to 4.2 pg/mL). And if you can – TSH levels should only be considered as a secondary parameter or metric. Some doctors and some thyroid experts now believe that TSH is pointless and serves no purpose once the diagnosis is determined (what does it really matter if you suppress it?). This elevation should only occur with VERY careful physician monitoring by your doctor looking for any potential side effects (palpitations, tachycardia, angina, MI, etc.)

Symptoms of Hypothyroidism and Benefits of Supplementation

What are the **symptoms/sequelae of hypothyroidism** and **benefits of T3/T4 supplementation**?

1. Subclinical hypothyroidism accompanying symptoms may include intolerance to cold, muscle cramps, dry skin, constipation, poor energy levels, fatigue and mental slowness[10].

2. LDL-C was higher in subjects with subclinical hypothyroidism[11].

3. Total cholesterol was higher in subjects with subclinical hypothyroidism[12].

4. Triglycerides were higher in subjects with subclinical hypothyroidism. Supplementing to optimal levels decreases triglyceride levels[13].

5. Supplementing with thyroid decreases total cholesterol and LDL-C[14].

6. Thyroid hormone does not cause weight loss but lends the energy to the patient sufficient for increased exercise that can lead to weight loss.

7. Hypothyroid patients can present with dyspnea on exertion, fatigue, and edema that may be the result of either pericardial effusion or CHF[15].

8. Most patients with CHF have hypothyroidism -- treating CHF with T3 (T3 was given IV in this study) improves cardiac output and vascular resistance[16].

9. Treating with combination therapy (T3 and T4) improves physical and mental well-being (vs. just giving T4), and to accomplish this, the study investigators optimized the serum Free T3 level[17].

10. Experts believe that even mild subclinical hypothyroidism[18] should be treated[19].

11. So-called subclinical hypothyroidism (Low T3 Syndrome for many endocrinologists) patients give many significant changes in a clinical symptom index (the Billewicz scale) in subclinical hypothyroid women (mean age, 50 years) compared with age-matched controls[20].

12. Subclinical hypothyroidism causes elevation in lipoprotein(a) levels increasing atherosclerosis[21]. *[This increases the deadly lipoprotein(a) so it's hard to rationalize why we let this occur when a cheap treatment option like this will clear that up.]*

13. Subclinical hypothyroidism causes significant alterations in memory and mood, including anxiety, depression, and somaticism, all of which return to normal with therapy with T4 AND T3[22].

14. Thyroxine replacement is actually NOT associated with risk of osteoporosis[23].

15. Women with diffuse hair loss? Try 1-3 grains of thyroid, push the dose a little and after 6 months or so they should have good hair regrowth. Comes out in clumps – very obvious – this is actually a telogen effluvium. Androgenic hair loss is very slow and occurs over a long period of time.

16. Hypothyroidism is associated with breast cancer in post-menopausal women[24]. If they are at some familial risk treat them aggressively.

17. Fibromyalgia can be treated with supraphysiologic doses of thyroid and most of

the time you will get good results if not total clearing of the symptoms[25]. This is due to a thyroid hormone resistance [26] or receptor failure so push the dose in these patients (within reason – monitor for potential serious side effects).

18. There is no lab test available to determine thyroid resistance (which appears to be multifactorial in nature), but from an extensive review of the literature receptor problems or even gross failure is much more common than anyone has perceived[27].

19. Synthroid® Rough Conversion Formula: On Synthroid® 0.1 mgm to 1.0 grains (60 mgm) of Armour®.

20. "I tend to treat everybody."[28]

–David S. Cooper, MD,

Director of the Division of Endocrinology,

Sinai Hospital of Baltimore, Maryland.

Her Hair Was Scraggly…(continued)

I looked at her labs – they'd only taken a few days to come back.

Her TSH was barely high. But still it was high. 5.1 UIU/ML

Her Free T3 (FT#) was super low – 1.6 PG/ML

And her Free T4 was low – 0.52 NG/DL

I looked at her. She was sitting quietly across from the desk. "Well, you're definitely hypothyroid." I slid her the copies of the reports. "I highlighted all the abnormals."

She laughed a little. "They're *all* abnormal."

"But just barely," I added.

She said, "That's what the last two doctors said – but neither one wanted to treat me."

"Why?"

"One said that because of my chronic constipation and stool softener intake I was bulimic and he didn't want to treat me with thyroid – even though my weight was fine."

"Uhh what?" I'd heard this kind of convoluted twisted reasoning before but it still always surprised me. But guilty as charged -- I guess I'd wondered too – when I was examining her thyroid for lumps and bumps I'd looked at her teeth and jaw, too – enamel was intact, jaw small -- she was not a purger, at least not that I was aware of. The stool softener thing had bugged me a little too but it fit with the thyroid. That doc had the right symptom, just the wrong root cause.

I shrugged and apologized for him, and didn't even know him, "Yeah, docs get a little twisted in their reasoning. It's how we are some times. I'm sure he meant well."

She nodded.

"But the question you should be asking is why? Why are you hypothyroid? Why is your thyroid not functioning well…" I looked at her in the face. "Got it? Someone needs to ask that."

"What do you mean?"
"Your TPO antibodies are not elevated so it's not Hashimoto's. Looking at your labs your pituitary is not reacting appropriately to the low thyroid. And also why is there low thyroid? None of it adds up."

She nodded, her brain working.

"Do you get muscle cramps? Charlie horses?"

She nodded again, bent over in her chair, and grabbed her leg – extending it a little. "At night – they're horrible and wake me up. Scares my husband to death."

I nodded. "Sounds like low magnesium and maybe zinc. We should start you on something for that but I want to get this intracellular vitamin and mineral panel blood test on you – looks at 39 different vitamins and minerals. It's very accurate. Takes four weeks to come back though. If you want you can come back and we'll go over the results."

She looked at me. "What about my thyroid?"

"We'll also start you on something now. We can always stop it in the future if it's really unnecessary."

She smiled. Feeling relief. "Whatever we need to do…"

16

I nodded.

"I want something natural… if possible."

"Nature-Throid® is an option and I usually prescribe that in situations like this. But I can put you on Synthroid®, too."

She shook her head no. "I heard about Synthroid® – no thanks. Nature-Throid® works."

"Okay, let's start at ¼ of a grain of Nature-Throid® -- and we'll have to go up from there. ¼ grain won't be enough and you'll definitely feel worse before you get better."

"What's a grain?"

"60 or 65 milligrams. 60 milligrams with Armour®. 65 milligrams is a grain with Nature-Throid® but *it does* come in ¼ grains (which are easier to adjust) and Armour® does not, so it's harder to adjust."

She nodded, understanding.

"Start on a ¼ grain a day the first week and go up ¼ grain a week. Stay at 1½ grains a day (six ¼ grains). You have to watch for side effects."

"And those are?"

"Jitters. Can't sleep. Heart racing and pounding. Nervousness. Promise me you'll call me ASAP on my cell phone if there's a problem." I slid my card forward – all my patients got it – they could call or text or email me anytime night or day. And some did. Most did not bother me ever.

17

She picked up and said a quiet thanks.

"Promise me…"

"I promise."

"Okay, let's draw your blood."

(To Be Continued)

CHAPTER 2

TRUE FACTS & MORE BENEFITS OF THYROID

1. Hypothyroidism increases with age[29].

2. The human thyroid system is almost identical to the porcine thyroid system[30] (so don't fret about the use of Armour® or NatureThroid®).

3. In the human system there are two main thyroid receptors:
    A. Deiodination receptors activate thyroid and convert from T4 to T3 (remember T3 is the active form of thyroid hormone).
    B. Nuclear retinoid receptors for thyroid are on all cells for thyroid hormone to function.

4. Similar to Type 2 Diabetes you can first get thyroid resistance [31] (also termed receptor exhaustion -- first felt to be genetic, we now know this is part of aging[32]) when either the deiodination receptor begins to fail or when the main peripheral retinoid receptors begin to fail[33]. When this happens, thyroid production and levels can rise in the bodies' attempt to overcome this resistance, plus the conversion of T4 to T3 is slowed.

5. According to one article the incidence of the syndromes of resistance to thyroid hormone is *unknown;* a limited survey suggested the

19

occurrence of 1 case in 50,000 live births[34] but by sheer reason and other studies looked at in this chapter, we must assume and know that thyroid receptor failure due to aging is *very common.*

6. T3 is the active moiety *at the cellular level* and much less common than T4 in the human body. T4 is inactive and is usually kept in reserve, while T3 is ten times more active and is, by all experts, considered the active thyroid hormone[35].

7. Remember the **symptoms of hypothyroidism**[36]:
   A. Fatigue
   B. Lower then normal body temperature
   C. Cold extremities
   D. Greater susceptibility to colds and other viruses (immunospression)
   E. Weight gain
   F. Depression
   G. Dry skin
   H. Headaches
   I. High cholesterol and other hyperlipidemias
   J. Inability of a female to get or maintain a pregnancy[37]

8. Thyroid resistance[38] occurs more often as we get older and is a recognized entity (not a false construct to benefit Armour®). This can be due to a number of reasons but thyroid receptor failure is the most common in the elderly despite many articles to the contrary. The usual cause of this "rare" disorder is felt to be genetic and the gene defect is also tied to insulin receptor failure[39].

9. Other than aging and genetics disorders, it is unclear as to why thyroid receptors fail and thyroid hormone resistance occurs. We would encourage more studies in this area but we suspect as in insulin receptor failure (i.e. insulin resistance) that testosterone and HGH probably assist in maintaining the viability of these receptors.

10. Like in diabetes, thyroid receptor activity, health, and longevity improvement occurs with HGH, which also improves end organ resistance. It is broadly believed that by giving HGH physiological amounts would be beneficial in thyroid resistance cases or when you suspect someone has failing receptors[40].

11. There are several versions of the deiodinated thyroid hormone beyond the T4 moiety – T3, T2, and T1 -- and all versions come with some activity in peripheral tissues (not just T3) though this activity has not yet been clearly defined in the literature. It is this activity that has led some researchers/practitioners to believe that some patients respond best to desiccated thyroid from the addition of these lesser-known, lesser-understood deiodinated thyroid hormones[41].

12. Because of this reason (#11) and others, desiccated porcine thyroid (Armour® Thyroid) is much preferable to synthetic T3 or T4 in almost all instances.

13. Knoll pharmaceutical who makes Synthroid® falsified some of their data in order to get

Synthroid® FDA approved and to be looked on more favorably by the medical community and physicians for some reason keep forgetting this. To support this contention:

"*Company Allegedly Hid Thyroid Research*," Brenda C. Coleman, Associated Press, April 16, 1997. This is where the story broke on Knoll *suppressing* the research allegedly showing that L-thyroxine was *less effective* than the cheaper alternatives (Armour® thyroid or its generics).

Also, from September 1997 -- according to what the FDA had placed in the **Federal register**, "*no currently marketed orally administered levothyroxine sodium product has been shown to demonstrate consistent potency and stability and, thus, no currently marketed orally administered levothyroxine sodium product is generally recognized as safe and effective.*"

14. There was a huge class action lawsuit in the 1990's against Knoll, which Knoll settled for an insignificant 87.4 million dollars, for this little bit of trickery.

15. The FDA has also told physicians that Armour® is safer and better than Synthroid® but we keep forgetting this. The United States Food and Drug Administration Letter to Synthroid® Manufacturer, Knoll Pharmaceuticals April 26, 2001, was a scathing response where the FDA officially denied Knoll's request, meaning that Synthroid® had to apply for a new drug

application by August of 2001 in order to remain legally on the market.

16. Even the CBS® show, **60 MINUTES®**, did a news article on television in the late 1990's for the public in regards to Knoll®.

17. Armour® is much cheaper than Synthroid®. (Generic is MUCH cheaper.)

18. The four main arguments against using desiccated porcine thyroid (Armour®) are bogus and not supported. We've all heard these. For example:

   A. "The desiccated *bovine* hormone is not even close to human thyroid so why give it?"

   FALSE.

   The formulation for decades has been PORCINE (pig) thyroid, and NOT bovine (cattle) and it is essentially identical. Regardless, the porcine thyroid IS molecularly identical to human.

   B. "Several years ago, researchers discovered that there was considerable variation in potency from batch to batch of the dessicated thyroid -- in short, a manufacturing quality issue."

   FALSE.

Dr. Purser and others before him have looked at this issue extensively, and *have not yet found any research that reported "considerable variation in potency from batch to batch."* But in the August 2001 letter from the FDA (noted above) that Synthroid® was denied because *it* could "not be Generally Recognized as Safe and Effective because it is of No Fixed Composition."

C. "Levothyroxine is safer and more potent so why give that weird animal thyroid?"

FALSE.

Here we go again. In 1997, the U.S. Food and Drug Administration issued a warning, via the **Federal Register**, that *"no currently marketed orally administered levothyroxine sodium product has been shown to demonstrate consistent potency and stability and, thus, no currently marketed orally administered levothyroxine sodium product is generally recognized as safe and effective."* (**Federal Register**, August 14, 1997)

D. "Angina or atrial fibrillation occurs more with desiccated thyroid."

FALSE.

These symptoms are much more common with excess L-thyroxine [42] (thus the FDA statement above in the **Federal Register**) but more rare with the healthy stew present in Armour® thyroid.

19. Giving the desiccated thyroid to patients allows them the healthy stew or milieu of T4, T3, T2, and T1 floating around in their system and they do have purposes[43]. Almost no doctor can tell you what T1 or T2 do but, they cannot also tell you what they do not do, or if they're even necessary. This is bad. Physicians should give it just to be safe since even the FDA believes desiccated animal thyroid is more or as safe then synthetic levothyroxine (if in doubt, see **Federal Register**, August 14, 1997).

20. The change in lab norms increased the number of Americans with thyroid illness from 13 million to approximately 27 million overnight in 2002! But our clinical experience has told us that even the major laboratories continue to give erroneous "normal ranges" for the tests, simply because they're not aware of the guidelines of the AACE or the information put out by their National Association of Clinical Biochemistry.

21. Now, 48 months after the new directives have been given, doctors are still largely unaware of these new lab guidelines for diagnosis and treatment. NOTICE TO ALL DOCTORS AND THEIR LABS! The TSH range has changed! The FDA also believes desiccated porcine thyroid is better and safer then synthetic T3! (Just in case you forgot again.) Regardless the

studies tend to ignore TSH and optimize T4 and T3 levels (the latter mainly because tell us why we should care if the inactive version of the hormone is optimized).

22. General myth on thyroid hormone prescribing (because of this myth it does not matter whether you are prescribing synthetic levothyroxine or desiccated porcine thyroid) goes like this, "Giving too much thyroid will suppress their pituitary and thyroid gland – this is a bad thing." That's right. Not really!

FALSE.

It is a bad thing to not give *enough* thyroid hormone but these patients will have had a naturally suppressed pituitary and thyroid anyway *before* you started them on thyroid (uhhh, that's why you decided to give them thyroid – remember?) – it's called aging. After you start them on thyroid supplementation you can check their free T4 but keep in mind if you check a TSH level it will probably be suppressed or low anyway. And that's all right because it will never come back unless you transplant them a new pituitary!

23. CoEnzyme Q10 is the last coenzyme in the energy pathway in the mitochondria of the cell and is inherently involved in the thyroid-energy pathways. If your patients are female or taking a little extra thyroid make absolutely sure you give them adequate amounts of a high quality CoEnzyme Q10 supplement [44] (200 mgm a day at least).

24. Taking adequate amounts of T4/T3 thyroid supplementation will cause:

A. Weight loss (WARNING: it is VERY illegal to prescribe for this purpose).

B. Lowered cholesterol and lipids[45].

C. Increased energy.

D. Warmer body temperature.

E. Increased immune resistance.

F. Increased cardiac output (decreased CHF)[46].

G. Increased hair and nail thickness.

H. Improved cardiac output[47].

I. No increased bone density loss (does not cause increased osteoporosis)[48].

J. Improved fertility (females)[49].

K. Clarity of thought and cognition improvements[50].

L. T4 is almost exclusively the hormone that passes through the blood brain barrier[51].

25. Some rare patients (usually women) have peripheral receptor sites (TR) that are not functioning nor binding the hormone properly so they will cheat and take massive doses of the thyroid hormone (9 to 15 grains a day!!!!). This will suppress the TSH level GREATLY so do not bother to get a TSH level on these patients. You will know who these are by the fact that they are very hyperactive and have lost a lot of weight. Make sure if you suspect someone's doing this that when you tell him or her to reduce their thyroid you also tell them to take a LOT (200 – 400 mg a day) of high quality CoEnzymeQ10 (CoQ10)[52].

26. ZINC sometimes helps! The peripheral T3 receptor is thought to require zinc to adopt its

biologically active conformation. Some of the effects of zinc deficiency, therefore, are due to loss of zinc from the T3 receptor and impairment of T3 action[53].

27. With excess exogenous or endogenous thyroid cardiac contractility and cardiac output are enhanced and systemic vascular resistance is decreased [54], while in hypothyroidism the opposite is true (you get increased vascular resistance, left ventricular hypertrophy)[55]. Which is better?

28. If you have a female patient who is incapable of getting pregnant or maintaining a pregnancy (and she's trying) and has tried everything check her thyroid – if in doubt, give her a mild dose (1/2 grain BID)[56].

29. Patients who take a combination of T4 and T3 (not just synthetic T4) have improved depression symptoms[57], feelings of well being, cardiac output, and quality of life – the goals of all worthwhile clinicians[58].

30. The psychiatric community has used T3 (Cytomel® - liothyronine) for years for mood stabilization, depression and mania with great effect and they rarely look at any lab work[59] and often usually use supraphysiologic doses.

31. If you have a patient with PCOS (Polycystic Ovary Syndrome) put them on thyroid supplementation and watch the great improvement[60].

32. You need to reassess all those chronic fatigue patients with odd annoying complaints that you historically have just hated seeing in your office – check their TSH, Free T3, and Free T4 with a high level of suspicion. If in doubt, act like a psychiatrist and put them on a little thyroid hormone (desiccated) anyway[61].

33. Too fatigued to exercise? Think of subclinical hypothyroidism[62].

34. Young and suffering from specific memory loss issues and feeling just generally lousy and seen numerous physicians without good effect? Try them on a low dose of desiccated thyroid[63]. And there is usually NO adverse effect to higher dose treatment[64]!!

35. Most cases of fibromyalgia fall into the category of type II (hormone resistant) hypothyroidism. Preliminary evidence suggests that serum hyaluronic acid is a simple, inexpensive, sensitive, and specific test that identifies fibromyalgia. The thyroid-resistant disorders might be treatable with *experimentally proven treatment of supraphysiologic doses of thyroid hormone.* Someone with total thyroid failure may have mild symptoms compared to someone who has moderate thyroid failure[65].

36. Know that the element selenium (200 mcg a day at most) assists the deiodinase enzyme in converting T4 to T3 (use if T4 is good but T3 is low). NOTE: Be careful – you can become toxic on selenium.

37. Recently, hypothyroidism has been associated as a risk factor for Bone, Skin and Breast cancers[66].

38. Even most of the experts think you should treat subclinical (read overt symptom free) hypothyroidism[67].

39. Overt symptoms of subclinical hypothyroidism include hypercholesterolemia, coronary disease, cerebrovascular disease, plus neuropsychiatric manifestations of mood depression, memory and cognition impairment and a declining sense of well being, and improves with both T4 and T3[68]. Why, as caregivers, would we not treat this?

40. Though endocrinologists claim it, TSH should not be used to evaluate the severity of thyroid failure. It's the free T3 hormone that affects the peripheral tissues at the cellular level[69] NOT the circulating TSH.

41. Rarely you will get a patient who's incredibly sensitive to any thyroid hormone[70] (despite lab and patient appearing as if hypothyroid) and they go into tachycardia or severe anxiety with the smallest doses. Just beware.

42. Remember -- treat the patient not the lab (unless level's are not optimized then give them a little extra)[71]. ☺

43. If you're treating with what you feel is adequate thyroid and their FT3 is 4.0 or thereabouts, and they still complain of cold and fatigue and exhaustion and hair loss –

consider that they may have thyroid resistance (also called RTH – Resistance to Thyroid Hormone). They may need to be given a higher dose. This is not new – has been known for centuries. Read up on it at the references attached[72] [73]. Here's a good book by Mark Starr, MD.

Her Hair Was Scraggly...(continued)

Her Spectracell™ Comprehensive Metabolic panel was back. And her hand was a little warmer, when I shook it. Not warm enough though.

We looked at the results.

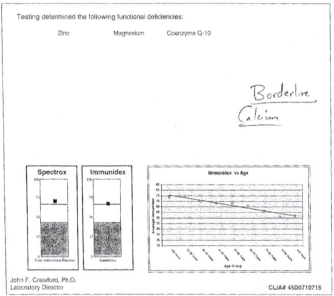

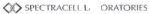

SpectraCell Laboratories, Inc.
Laboratory Test Report

Accession Number:

Repletion Suggestions

1. Zinc	25 mg daily
2. Magnesium	150 mg b.i.d. (300 mg daily) as aspartate, citrate, lysinate, glycinate, or malate
3. Coenzyme Q-10	100 mg daily of CoQ10 Take each dose with a meal

Please note: Supplementation is usually required for four to six months to effect the repletion of a functional deficiency in lymphocytes

Suggestions for supplementation with specific micronutrients must be evaluated and approved by the attending physician. This decision should be based upon the clinical condition of the patient and the evaluation of the effects of supplementation on current treatment and medication of the patient.

SpectraCell Laboratories, Inc.
Laboratory Test Report

Accession Number:

Micronutrients	Patient Results (% Control)	Functional Abnormals	Reference Range (greater than)
B Complex Vitamins			
Vitamin B1 (Thiamin)	100		>78%
Vitamin B2 (Riboflavin)	71		>53%
Vitamin B3 (Niacinamide)	105		>80%
Vitamin B6 (Pyridoxine)	72		>54%
Vitamin B12 (Cobalamin)	19		>14%
Folate	48		>32%
Pantothenate	15		>7%
Biotin	51		>34%
Amino Acids			
Serine	53		>30%
Glutamine	57		>37%
Asparagine	46		>39%
Metabolites			
Choline	32		>20%
Inositol	73		>58%
Carnitine	61		>46%
Fatty Acids			
Oleic Acid	73		>65%
Other Vitamins			
Vitamin D3 (Cholecalciferol)	67		>50%
Vitamin A (Retinol)	81		>70%
Vitamin K2	61		>30%
Minerals			
Calcium	40		>38%
Manganese	68		>50%
Zinc	37	Deficient	>37%
Copper	51		>42%
Magnesium	35	Deficient	>37%
Carbohydrate Metabolism			
Glucose-Insulin Interaction	44		>38%
Fructose Sensitivity	50		>34%
Chromium	48		>40%
Antioxidants			
Glutathione	56		>42%
Cysteine	50		>41%
Coenzyme Q-10	86	Deficient	>86%
Selenium	82		>74%
Vitamin E (A-tocopherol)	93		>84%
Alpha Lipoic Acid	88		>81%
Vitamin C	53		>40%
SPECTROX™			
Total Antioxidant Function	71		>40%
Proliferation Index			
Immunidex	65		>40%

The reference ranges listed in the above table are valid for male and female patients 12 years of age or older.

I carefully explained to her how her intracellular deficiency showed the perfect storm – except for no selenium deficiency, she had all the deficiencies that could most effect thyroid production and the thyroid (FT3) receptors – causing thyroid resistance. Plus I explained how these vitamin deficiencies were going to leave her feeling incredibly exhausted ALL THE TIME.

She looked at me. "All the time?"

"Plus cause leg cramps – the kind of screamers that wake up at night screaming."

She chuckled.

"On top of all that they can and will affect your thyroid receptors – picture these as tiny little complex engines or machines on the cell surface where the T3 plugs in. These are critical parts of those engines and without them they'll fail. You need them to work or you get thyroid resistance."

"What's that? Thyroid resistance?"

"It's like insulin resistance but it's where the thyroid hormone does not work like it should because the receptor or tiny engine is dysfunctional or broken. In insulin resistance, doctors will give more insulin to overcome the insulin receptor being dysfunctional – I mean it functions occasionally and so you need lots of T3 around it to plug into it when it achieves it's rare position of function. That's why we may need to elevate your T3 levels a little to make it work but we'll see. Plus all this could explain your hair loss and alopecia."

I showed her a study. "It's the zinc deficiency causing the hair loss or alopecia – I see this often."

© Freund Publishing House Ltd., London

Journal of Pediatric Endocrinology & Metabolism, 22, 1075-1081 (2009)

Alopecia: Association with Resistance to Thyroid Hormones

Tulay Guran[1], Rifat Bircan[2], Serap Turan[1] and Abdullah Bereket[1]

[1]Department of Pediatric Endocrinology and Diabetes, Marmara University Hospital, Istanbul and
[2]Namık Kemal University, Division of Biology, Department of Molecular Biology and Genetics,
Faculty of Arts and Sciences, Tekirdag, Turkey

ABSTRACT

Resistance to thyroid hormone (RTH) syndrome is caused by thyroid hormone β receptor (TRβ) mutations. Goiter, learning disabilities, psychological abnormalities, sinus tachycardia, hearing deficits, short stature, and growth delay are among the most common symptoms in patients with RTH. Alopecia areata (AA) ,is an autoimmune disease of the hair follicle, frequently associated with other autoimmune disorders. In some cases local alopecia of different genetic backgrounds could be misdiagnosed as AA. We describe here clinical, biochemical and genetic features of a family having RTH syndrome, caused by a novel TRβ mutation, coexistent with alopecia. Mutational analyses of the TRβ gene and the hairless gene (HR) in genomic DNA were performed. The index patient is a 9-$^5/_{12}$ year-old boy with RTH due to a novel heterozygous missense mutation of the TRβ gene (I353V), and diffuse, patchy alopecia without autoimmune thyroid disease. This mutation was also detected in his father and elder brother, who also have local alopecia. One of his paternal aunts and paternal grandmother have local alopecia and they have previously been operated for goiter. Although they refused any genetic analysis, the pre-operative medical report of the paternal aunt was compatible with RTH. A second paternal aunt has alopecia totalis universalis but has no RTH mutation in genomic DNA. Genomic DNA sequence of the HR gene of the family (index patient, two brothers, father, mother and second paternal aunt) was normal as well.

Conclusion: We speculate that RTH due to a novel I353V TRβ mutation could be causally related to different phenotypic expressions of alopecia in this family, either by a direct effect of unresponsiveness to T3 of the hair follicle or by the modulated action of the HR gene.

KEY WORDS

thyroid hormone receptor beta (TRβ) mutation, resistance to thyroid hormone, alopecia, hairless gene, alopecia totalis universalis

INTRODUCTION

Resistance to thyroid hormone (RTH) is an autosomal dominant disorder (except the first case described by Refetoff et al. which was inherited recessively[3]) that leads to elevated free thyroid hormone levels in the presence of normal or increased serum thyroid-stimulating hormone (TSH) concentrations. Estimated incidence of RTH is 1/40,000 live births[2]. RTH, despite a variable severity in clinical presentation, is generally characterized by the absence of the usual symptoms and metabolic consequences of thyroid hormone excess. Goiter, learning disabilities, psychological abnormalities, sinus tachycardia, hearing deficits, short stature, growth delay are among the most common symptoms in patients with RTH[1,4]. The severity of the hormonal resistance is dependent on the feature and expression of the underlying mutation. This mutation is mostly in one allele of the thyroid hormone receptor β (TRβ) gene. To date, in about 2,000 cases belonging to approxi-

Reprint address:
Tulay Guran
Department of Pediatric Endocrinology
Marmara University Medical Hospital
Tophanelioglu Caddesi No. 13/15
81190 Altunizade Istanbul, Turkey
e-mail: tulayguran@yahoo.com

"Any problems with taking that thyroid?"

"No."

"Are you any warmer?"

"Yes. Especially my feet and hands."

"Let me give you a list of vitamins and let's check your thyroid levels. I'll call you with the results so you can adjust accordingly. I suspect you're still not on enough. And it will take ninety days on the vitamins to correct those deficiencies – they didn't happen overnight."

"And I'll feel even better?"

I nodded. "Pretty quickly but ninety days to feel solid. Let's check your blood and get that going then I can suggest some vitamins. We'll recheck levels in ninety days when we repeat your SpectraCell™."

She smiled as we stood – we had a lot of work to do.

(To Be Continued)

CHAPTER 3

MONITORING AND CHECKING LEVELS

This might be a paradigm shift for you in thyroid care and thought. Good!

Forget everything you know about thyroid problems and start over. Know that TSH levels have zero impact on the way a patient feels.

Critical Point #1: Treat the patient's clinical symptoms FIRST not their lab. Remember that we're "clinicians" and not "labicians." The lab levels serve only as a guide, but you have to use your brain to interpret them correctly.

Critical Point #2: Your patient's symptoms stem from the level of Free T3[74] (or lack thereof) in their system – not from their level of TSH or T4[75].

Critical Point #3: Look first and mainly at your patient's Free T3 levels[76].

Critical Point #4: A low but normal level of Free T3 is clinically significantly low, especially because most patients will also have concurrent symptoms of fatigue and lethargy. From another perspective that Free T3 level is really lower than it appears because most of these patients have additional T3 receptor failure on their peripheral tissues[77].

Critical Point #5: If your patient's Free T3 levels are normal and they still have symptoms of hypothyroidism think thyroid T3 receptor failure on peripheral cells. This is a common finding in the elderly and people with chronic illnesses[78] such as chronic renal failure (CKD) and they can have low T3 and T4 levels with normal thyroid-stimulating hormone (TSH) levels[79].

Critical Point #6: Don't be afraid to optimize their level of Free T3 to 3.9-4.0 pg/ml or above. If they have receptor failure they may need this extra exogenous T3 and T4[80] to feel well[81]. (Always watch for or ask about cardiac problems *before* doing so though.)

Critical Point #7: A small percentage of hypothyroid patients will have thyroid sensitivity in their hypothyroidism making their cardiac tissue exquisitely sensitive to any level of thyroid causing atrial fibrillation[82], SVTs, angina, and other cardiac abnormalities. Start these patients on a tiny dose (1/4 grain of desiccated thyroid) twice a day to begin with.

Critical Point #8: Remember if they have also any thyroid 2'deiodinase[83] (D2) failure or malfunction (not uncommon in the elderly) they will not convert a significant amount of exogenous or endogenous T4 to the active hormone (T3)[84], no matter how much synthetic T4 (levo-thyroxine) you or their endocrinologist gives them, thus their T3 levels will remain low or low normal, while their Free T4 will remain very high and their TSH may be suppressed or elevated. Remember – look at the Free T3 level first and mainly!

Critical Point #9: MALPRACTICE WARNING! If all their levels are very low (Free T3, Free T4 and TSH) and they're acting goofy or psychotic BE VERY CAREFUL – these patients have an emergent mixedematous coma and need to be admitted to the hospital. You will treat these patients with kid gloves very slowly and carefully because they are extremely sensitive to thyroid hormone (starting them on ¼ grain a day of desiccated thyroid and only increasing it every 4 or 5 days).

In general, check a TSH, Free Serum T4, and Free Serum T3 (always focusing on the Free T3 level) to begin with when you first evaluate the patient. Remember that a relatively low or normal free T4 and free T3 with a low TSH can indicate a thyroid inadequacy.

After optimizing therapies you can check their Free T3, but keep in mind if you check a TSH level, it will probably be suppressed (this is alright because you've optimized their thyroid levels).

CHAPTER 4

THYROID PRACTICE GEMS

A. Choice of product can vary but most of my patients want the most natural they can get so I tend to prescribe NatureThroid®(prescribed in grains like Armour).

B. Or order it from your compounding pharmacy by saying on the script: Compounded T3/T4 Capsule (Armour® formula)

C. Start low (1/2 to 1 grain per day) of the desiccated natural form of thyroid (an encapsulated forms works best).

D. 1 Grain of Armour = 60 mgm, however 1 Grain of NatureThroid = 65mg

E. Do not try to use a sustained release thyroid or you will get unusually low levels despite treatment with even larger doses.

F. Average daily dose is about 2 grains in males and 3 grains in females.

G. If they have RTH (Resistance to Thyroid Hormone due to faulty receptors) don't be fooled by a low TSH. As a matter of fact it is pointless (and confusing) to continue to check TSH levels in these patients. Just give them more desiccated thyroid until symptoms resolve. MONITOR for SIDE EFFECTS!

H. Never ever give thyroid for weight loss (even though weight normalization tends to occur when the dose is appropriate) – this is illegal.

I. NOTE: MALPRACTICE WARNING! Always watch for angina or CAD or SVT arrhythmia problems in these patients. Could be from too much thyroid or paradoxically even too little thyroid.

CHAPTER 5

WHY IS FREE T4 IMPORTANT?

Free T4 or levo-thyroxine, though it's treated like the red headed stepchild, is critical. Why is this? It's because peer reviewed studies[85] have shown us it's the *only* thyroid hormone (T3 does not) that passes through the blood-brain-barrier[86] (BBB) and keeps your brain fired up.

A low FT4 means brain fog and brain fatigue like crazy.

CHAPTER 6

VITAMINS AND MINERALS

FOR THYROID FUNCTION

CoEnzyme Q10 Capsules

If you give thyroid then always give CoEnzyme Q10[87] along with it, especially in patients who have CHF and *especially* in patients taking a statin[88].

Why?

CoQ10 is the last co-enzyme in the energy pathway (the Kreb's Cycle or Citric Acid Cycle) and is critical to energy levels.

If you're tired all the time yet your doctor is always telling you your thyroid levels are good then you better add CoQ10 – here's the kind I take -- Qunol™ and it's available at Amazon™. I take two per day unless a fatigue wall hits then I'll throw down five.

I also like (and helped design, but get no money from it) YLEO's Omegagize3™ at four per day.

Iodine Capsules

I've seen only one patient who improved taking iodine.

But here's a statistic that I am not sure I believe -- in

the US, it's estimated that one in seven women suffers from iodine deficiency.[89]

"Many people don't know that flour isn't iodized anymore, and iodization of salt is still voluntary in the US — only one-fifth of our salt is actually iodized. In reading further, I've found that we're trending back toward iodine deficiency. Iodine intake has declined 50% in North America in the past 30–40 years, and this is consistent with what I'm seeing in my patients.

As recently as 2004, the New England Journal of Medicine defined our iodine status here in the US as "marginal," based on data acquired from the International Council for the Control of Iodine Deficiency Disorder and the World Health Organization (WHO). More specifically, the WHO data suggest the greater risk in the US is not iodine deficiency per se, but iodine-induced hyperthyroidism (overproduction of thyroid hormones) or iodine-induced hypothyroidism. Interestingly, both these problems can occur when people who are already iodine-deficient are given too much iodine, too quickly. I believe practitioners need to proceed more cautiously when prescribing iodine supplements, slowly bringing levels up rather than overloading right up front. (More on our treatment protocol for iodine deficiency below). But the WHO perspective seems to confirm that iodine deficiency does exist here in the US.[90]"

Why Has Iodine Disappeared?

"In addition to iodine's disappearance from our food supply, exposure to toxic competing halogens (bromine, fluorine, chlorine and perchlorate) has dramatically increased.

You absorb these halogens through your food, water, medications and environment, and they selectively occupy your iodine receptors, further deepening your iodine deficit.

Fluoridation of water is a major contributor to iodine deficiency, besides being very damaging to your health in many other ways.

Additional factors contributing to falling iodine levels are:

- Diets low in fish, shellfish and seaweed
- Vegan and vegetarian diets
- Decreased use of iodized salt
- Less use of iodide in the food and agricultural industry

Use of radioactive iodine in many medical procedures, which competes with natural iodine."[91]

Bromides Are a Problem for Iodine, Too

"Bromides are a menace to your endocrine system and are present all around you.

Despite a ban on the use of potassium bromate in flour by the World Health Organization, bromides can still be found in some over-the-counter medications, foods, and personal care products.

The use of potassium bromate as an additive to commercial breads and baked goods has been a huge contributor to bromide overload in Western cultures.

Sodium bromate can be found in products such as permanent waves, hair dyes, and textile dyes.

Benzylkonium is used as a preservative in some cosmetics. Even trace amounts of bromine can trigger severe acne in sensitive individuals. And who needs skin care products that cause acne?

Bromine is also found in fire retardants used in carpets, mattresses, upholstery, and furniture and some medical equipment.

Based on animal research, bromides have been linked to behavioral changes and neurodevelopmental disorders, including Attention Deficit Disorders, in children.

The United States is quite behind in putting an end to the egregious practice of allowing bromine chemicals in your foods and products whereas other nations have taken the bull by the horns:

- In 1990, the United Kingdom banned bromate in bread
- In 1994, Canada did the same
- Brazil recently outlawed bromide in flour products
- The European Union has banned some PBDE compounds (polybrominated diphenyl ethers)

What's taking us in the states so long?

Again, corporate profits trump health concerns when it comes to doing what is best for the public."[92]

Getting Your Iodine Levels Up

"If you are iodine deficient, I recommend adding sea vegetables to your diet.

The best source of organically bound iodine that I know of is non-commercially harvested seaweeds. The dose is about 5 grams a day or about one ounce per week, so a pound would last about two months.

It is typically better to obtain a nutrient from a natural food whenever possible than from a supplement, so use supplements only as a last resort.

Some patients also report that they respond better to food-based forms of iodine -- like seaweeds -- than the supplement forms. However, if you are going to use a supplement I would strongly advise using supersaturated iodine (SSKI) which is available as an inexpensive prescription. Typically 1-3 drops a day are all that are required.

Please avoid using Lugol's solution or iodine, as that can actually worsen your thyroid condition.
The fact that your thyroid only transports iodine in its ionized form (i.e. iodide) is straight out of the textbooks. Your thyroid reduces iodide (I-) into iodine (I2) for use in formation of thyroglobulin. Your body doesn't utilize iodine directly. It has to split the I2 into two I- ions, which is an oxidative reaction that causes oxidative stress.

Iodide transporters are located in other areas of your body besides the thyroid gland, including your breasts and colon. One family of iodide transporters is called the sodium-iodide symporter, and the other is called pendren. Dr. David Brownstein (see below) discusses the sodium-iodide symporter but doesn't mention pendren. However like all ion transporters they too require a charge in order to move a molecule across the membrane, which means iodine, must be in its ionized form.

It's possible that some may see good results using Lugol's for some afflictions, but according to autism expert Catherine Tamara, in her experience it is very clear that children with autism, and their mothers, do fine with iodide, but not necessarily with iodine."[93]

For Iodine Deficiency Disorder and the subsequent goiter, take iodine capsules to alleviate [94]. This situation can also cause either subclinical or overt hypothyroidism so test accordingly.

The best iodine capsules at the correct dose that I use are on Amazon™.

Otherwise take iodide, like this Solaray™ iodide capsule.

Selenium Capsules

Selenium is not only critical to the manufacture of thyroid hormone in the gland but to the functionality of the thyroid receptor site, and more important is integral to the deiodinase enzyme [95] that removes iodine off T4 so it can become T3 (the active form of the thyroid hormone).

A deficiency will seriously impede both and make you appear or feel (because of thyroid dysfunction [96]) hypothyroid when you are not.

Take this at 200 mcg to supplement. You can get a good dose and brand here through my affiliate site connecting to Amazon™.

BEWARE on selenium as you can become toxic on it so only take a bottle every other year or so and if in doubt get your levels checked.

Selenium Toxicity

"Although selenium is an essential trace element, it is toxic if taken in excess. Exceeding the Tolerable Upper Intake Level of 400 micrograms per day can lead to selenosis.

This 400 microgram Tolerable Upper Intake Level is based primarily on a 1986 study of five Chinese patients who exhibited overt signs of selenosis and a follow up study on the same five people in 1992.

The 1992 study actually found the maximum safe dietary Se intake to be approximately 800 micrograms per day (15 micrograms per kilogram body weight), but suggested 400 micrograms per day to not only avoid toxicity, but also to avoid creating an imbalance of nutrients in the diet and to account for data from other countries.

The Chinese people who suffered from selenium toxicity ingested selenium by eating corn grown in extremely selenium-rich stony coal (carbonaceous shale).

This coal was shown to have selenium content as high as 9.1%, the highest concentration in coal ever recorded in literature. A dose of selenium as small as 5 mg per day can be lethal for many humans.

Symptoms of selenosis include a garlic odor on the breath, gastrointestinal disorders, hair loss, sloughing of nails, fatigue, irritability, and neurological damage.

Extreme cases of selenosis can result in cirrhosis of the liver, pulmonary edema, and death. Elemental selenium and most metallic selenides have relatively low toxicities because of their low bioavailability.

By contrast, selenates and selenites are very toxic, having an oxidant mode of action similar to that of arsenic trioxide[97]."

Zinc Tablets

Like selenium, zinc is not only critical to the manufacture of thyroid hormone in the gland but to the functionality of the thyroid receptor site (specifically the T3 receptor[98]).

A deficiency will seriously impede both and make you appear hypothyroid when you are not. I've seen this dozens of times – back to going primitive, diving deeper and getting intracellular vitamin panels.

Zinc deficiencies will also cause severe hair loss in women along with their pseudo-hypothyroidism. Often this is diagnosed as alopecia[99]. Just beware of it.

Here's a good zinc supplement on Amazon™.

Her Hair Was Scraggly...(continued)

It took ten days for her thyroid profile to come back. I faxed it to her and we Facetimed™.

"How are you feeling?"

"Better," she said. "Not as tired and it's very nice. My hair is not coming out in handfuls any more."

"Good. Leg cramps gone yet?

"No, had a bad one the other night. My leg *still* hurts from it."

"Yep, I've had that too – those are *HORRIBLE* – it takes like 87 to 90 days to go away – and then you feel really good."

She nodded – her image on my Macbook™ going in and out of focus. "How's my thyroid?"

"Your Free T3 is still too low. It's at 2.6. Waaaay too low still."

"Where do I want that?"

"Closer to 4.0. Like the GPA you probably had in college."

She said, "Not quite. Maybe you did..."

"Your FT4 is at 0.72. I like it above 1.0. Free T4 passes through the BBB – the blood brain barrier – helps clear out brain fog. Free T3 does not go into the brain."

"With Nature-Throid™ will that go up?"

"Yep. Why don't you slowly go up two more doses of the ¼ grain and then let's re-check levels. But stop if you have any side effects. Wait at least a week between dose increases."

"Okay, when will we re-check?"

"In four weeks."

She nodded and we ended the call. But her advancement was good. It was as good as could be expected.

(To Be Continued)

CHAPTER 7

ESSENTIAL OILS THAT

SUPPORT THYROID FUNCTION

SINGLE ESSENTIAL OILS
Myrtle Essential Oil[100]

"Do you have myrtle essential oil in your medicine cabinet? How about in your kitchen cupboard? This essential oil can help your family's health in many ways.

Myrtle (Myrtus communis L., Myrtaceae) is a medicinal herb that is used in traditional medicine in many parts of the world. Its berries, leaves and fruits have been used extensively as a traditional folk medicine for the treatment of disorders such as diarrhea, peptic ulcer, hemorrhoids, inflammation, pulmonary and skin diseases. Clinical and experimental research studies suggest that the essential oil of myrtle possesses an even broader range of benefits, which include antioxidative, anticancer, anti-diabetic, antiviral, antibacterial, and antifungal properties. It also protects the liver (hepatoprotective) and the nervous system (neuroprotective)[101].

Myrtus communis *[common myrtle],* is a native shrub in the Middle East. It grows in all the countries that border the Mediterranean. Countries where myrtle is native include: Turkey, Morocco, Algeria, Tunisia, France, Spain, Greece, and Italy. It has been brought to southern Britain and southern France.

The oil can be extracted from the leaves, branches, and berries. The oil that is most commonly used medicinally is extracted from the leaves. This oil will be liquid at room temperature. The color will range from clear to greenish-yellow to yellow-very-light-orange. Its aroma is reminiscent of frankincense or bay. Some examples of myrtle oil have a slight hint of camphor or eucalyptus. The oil from the myrtle berries is used as a flavoring for drinks and alcoholic beverages throughout the Mediterranean Area.

The name "myrtle" is also used for several other unrelated plants commonly found in the United States. These unrelated plants are called crepe myrtle, wax myrtle, and creeping myrtle."

Myrtle Oil Normalizes the functioning of the Thyroid and Ovaries

Dr. David Stewart describes the amazing way that the human body and this essential oil work together to promote thyroid health.

(Myrtus communis) is an adaptogen that can stimulate an increase or a decrease in thyroid activity depending on a person's condition. Drugs are incapable of such intelligent discriminations and act only in preprogrammed directions, like robots, whether beneficial or not[102].

Daniel Penoel, M.D. of France for normalizing hormonal imbalances of the thyroid and ovaries, has researched myrtle oil. It also has benefits for decongesting the respiratory system and the sinuses[103].

Adaptogen: an adaptogen will increase the functioning of a gland when its functioning is low, or will lower an overactive gland. The same oil will bring the functioning of the gland to a more normal state whether it is underfunctioning or overfunctioning.

CHAPTER 8

HASHIMOTO'S THYROIDITIS

It drives me crazy how so many patients say they have Hashimoto's disease.

My thought (and not being rude here) is, so? That's great their doc made that diagnosis but how'd they treat it and did that treat it adequately?

DIAGNOSIS

The diagnosis is simple (from the Mayo Clinic website[104]):

"Diagnosis of Hashimoto's disease is based on your signs and symptoms and the results of blood tests that measure levels of thyroid hormone and thyroid-stimulating hormone (TSH) produced in the pituitary gland. These may include:

A hormone test.

Blood tests can determine the amount of hormones produced by your thyroid and pituitary glands. If your thyroid is underactive, the level of thyroid hormone is low. At the same time, the level of TSH is elevated because your pituitary gland tries to stimulate your thyroid gland to produce more thyroid hormone.

An antibody test.

Because Hashimoto's disease is an autoimmune disorder, the cause involves production of abnormal antibodies. A blood test may confirm the presence of antibodies against thyroid peroxidase (TPO antibodies), an enzyme normally found in the thyroid gland that plays an important role in the production of thyroid hormones."

LAB EXAMPLES

Blood Tests	* 24.01.2011	* 16.07.2011	* 24.08.2011	* 20.01.2012		
Thyroid						
TSH	* 7.55	* 45.3	* 0.39	* <0.0005	mU/L	0.40 - 4.00
Free T4	13.9	* 7.6	* 19.3	* 20.1	pmol/L	9.0 - 19.0
Free T3		* 2.1	5.2	* 5.8	pmol/L	2.6 - 6.00
Thyroglobulin Ab				* 255	IU/mL	0-80
Thyroid Peroxidase Ab				* >1000	IU/mL	0-120
Iron						
Ferritin	* 7	* 23		72	ug/L	30 - 300
Iron		14.7		9.5	umol/L	5.0 - 30.0
transferrin		3.1		2.4	g/L	2.0 - 3.2
TIBC (Calc)		68		54	umol/L	46 - 70
Saturation		22		18	%	10 - 45

TREATMENT

It is usually not treated adequately in the patients who end up at my office (they've discovered the "HALF MEASURE" thing of which so many doctors are guilty) but I'm sure in the vast majority of patients it must be (or there are millions of miserable people out there). For some reason the proper treatment of Hashimoto's thyroiditis *appears* to be mysterious and really complicated.

Here's news for everyone:

IT IS NOT HARD.

This book has really been the discussion of treating this disease especially.

From the Mayo Clinic website[105] (they like to keep it simple too): "Hashimoto's disease is a condition in which your immune system attacks your thyroid, a small gland at the base of your neck below your Adam's apple. The thyroid gland is part of your endocrine system, which produces hormones that coordinate many of your body's activities.

The resulting inflammation from Hashimoto's disease, also known as chronic lymphocytic thyroiditis, often leads to an underactive thyroid gland (hypothyroidism). Hashimoto's disease is the most common cause of hypothyroidism in the United States. It primarily affects middle-aged women but also can occur in men and women of any age and in children.

Doctors test your thyroid function to help detect Hashimoto's disease. *Treatment of Hashimoto's disease with thyroid hormone replacement usually is simple and effective.*"

Read that last sentence again. They did not say "Treatment of Hashimoto's disease with thyroid hormone replacement usually is COMPLICATED and INEFFECTIVE." They said, *"replacement usually is simple and effective."*

So to keep it simple and effective and track your Free T3 and Free T4.

That's it.

Who cares if you suppress the TSH? It's absolutely ineffective because the thyroid has been turned into swiss cheese by your antibodies so if you suppress it what does it matter?

Her Hair Was Scraggly…(continued)

Her second Spectracell™ Comprehensive Metabolic panel was back plus her hand, when I shook it, was hot and almost sweaty. She had her hair in a pony – but it still looked noticeably thicker to me.

"How you feeling?"

"Good. Really good. Solid now."

"Nice – well your Spectracell™ was completely clear. And your last Free T3 was 3.8. Your Free T4 was 1.1. All perfect."
She smiled, "Well I feel it. My hair is coming in super thick."

I nodded and smiled. "I can see that – still hiding it in the pony tail though."

She smiled. "Yes, I guess I can quit doing that." She looked at me. "So where do we go from here?"

"Keep on your current dose and vitamins. Then let's check you in three to four months."

She nodded.

"Then later, after you're stable, you can come in once a year."

She nodded. "Thanks. And thank you for figuring all this out. This has been remarkable. Saved my life."

"Whatever." I smiled. "Any doc could have done this."

"If you say so…"

"See you in three to four months."

She nodded and I smiled.

(To Be Continued)

CHAPTER 9

GRAVE'S DISEASE

Grave's disease is where your eyes bug out horribly from an unknown cause – yep, though it's felt to be autoimmune, researchers never have figured out what causes this disorder. There are also some other symptoms and signs of Grave's Disease – of course these are signs and symptoms of hyperthyroidism which include irritability, muscle weakness, sleeping problems, a fast heartbeat, poor tolerance of heat, diarrhea, and weight loss. Other symptoms may include thickening of the skin on the shins, known as pretibial myxedema, and eye problems such as bulging, a condition known as Graves' ophthalmopathy [106]. This is actually an ophthalmopathy – and selenium has been shown to help[107] a little.

But seriously – this is such a bad problem (and potentially permanent) that you have to get into to see an ophthalmologist ASAP when you have this or the damage will stay.

You get a permanent proptosis and lid retraction as in this picture so please get it treated!

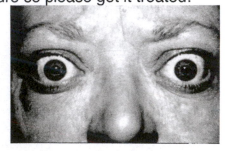

CHAPTER 10

REVERSE T3 – WHAT IT MEANS

(Borrowed from an amazing thyroid website to which everyone should go -- http://www.stopthethyroidmadness.com/reverse-t3/)

"A healthy thyroid produces the following hormones: T4, T3, T2, T1 and calcitonin. T4, a storage hormone and the most abundant, is meant to convert to T3, the most active hormone. T3 is also made directly.

But there's another substance produced by the thyroid called RT3, which stands for Reverse T3, and it comes from the conversion of the storage hormone T4. And it's NORMAL to have RT3.

Why does anyone produce RT3 (Reverse T3)?

Your body, especially the liver, can constantly be converting T4 to RT3 as a way to get rid of any unneeded T4. In any given day, it's stated that 40% of T4 goes to T3 and 20% of T4 goes to Reverse T3.

But in any situation where your body needs to conserve energy and focus on something else, it will change the above percentages, changing the conversion of RT3 to 50% or more, and the T3 goes down, down. Examples are emotional, physical, or biological stress, such as being chronically or acutely sick (the flu, pneumonia, etc), after surgery, after a car accident or any acute injury, chronic stress causing high cortisol, being exposed to an extremely cold environment, diabetes, aging, or even being on drugs like beta blockers and amiodarone. But there's

65

another reason for thyroid patients. Read on.

What specifically are the reasons I, as a thyroid patient, make too much RT3?

On top of the chronic stresses of your life, there are three common physiological reasons patients have noted, with the first two related to your adrenals (low cortisol, high cortisol), and the third related to your iron levels. Even low B12 and other chronic inflammation and other health issues can cause it.

When biological stress is excessive, such as being on the inadequate treatment of T4-only or being held hostage to the lousy TSH lab test (both which keep you underdosed or hypo), your adrenal glands produce high amounts of cortisol to help you cope with ongoing hypothyroidism and lingering symptoms and conditions. The excess cortisol inhibits the conversion of T4 to T3, and instead produces even larger amounts of RT3, creating an RT3 problem.

When biological stress is ongoing, your adrenals will eventually produce less cortisol (aka "adrenal fatigue" or "adrenal insufficiency"), dropping from high cortisol to a mix of high and low, the to all low. And those low levels can cause chronic anxiety, poor coping skills, paranoia, easy nausea, sensitivity to light or sounds, psychological issues, etc. When you don't make enough cortisol, thyroid hormones can pool high in your blood. So your body responds by converting the T4 to excess RT3.

When iron goes low, which is quite common in thyroid patients due to low stomach acid, your red blood cells become less plentiful (or you have enough, but they are weak and pale), and carrying thyroid hormones via your blood becomes inadequate, causing thyroid hormones to pool in your blood. The body responds by producing excessive amounts of RT3 to clear out the excess T4.

***Note that you can have either an iron problem, or a cortisol problem, or BOTH. There are other reasons you have high RT3, such as the excess inflammation and more, but the above are quite common and worthy to explore first.

Can lab work help me discover this? What do I look for?

First, you have room to be suspicious when your Free T4 is higher in the range for awhile, especially above 1.4, and your free T3 is lower. Even having a high Free T3 due to adrenal or iron problems (see below) can be the beginning of too much RT3. But doing the RT3 has given patients the best clue, especially looking at the ratio between it and the FT3.

With the RT3 labwork, you are not necessarily looking for a Reverse T3 result high in the range, though that in itself can be a good clue. Instead, you are looking for a problem in the ratio between the RT3 and the Free T3. i.e dividing the Free T3 by the Reverse T3 (Free T3 ÷ RT3)...though they need to be in the same measurement. See the I hate math heading below). For healthy amounts of RT3, The ratio result should be 20 or larger. If lower, you may have a problem. Janie has noted that many patients without an excess RT3 issue have a result of 23 or 24.

One place patients gained good information about all the above was from Dr. Kent Holtorf. If you scroll down on the former page, you'll also see mention of a study done with elderly men and RT3. Additionally, in the study article titled "Reverse T3 is the best measurement of thyroid tissue levels" found in the 2005, volume 90 issue of The Journal of Clinical Endocrinology & Metabolism, it states that "the T3/rT3 ratio is the most useful marker for tissue hypothyroidism and as a marker of diminished cel-lular functioning."

If you use the total T3, you are looking for a ratio greater than 10. If lower, you have a problem. Note that the unit of measurements for the RT3 and Free T3 are often different on your labwork and will need to be changed in order to be the same. Figuring out your ratio is here.

Can I order my own labwork for this, since I doubt my doctor will do this?

To order your own labwork, go to my home page and use the DirectLabs™ link. Remember to order a free T3 at the same time for ratio comparison. All facilities can test your ferritin without a doctor's prescription.

I hate math. How can I figure out my ratio?

If you don't feel very math-savvy, STTM has created a beta conversion method for you, here. It still has a few kinks in places we are trying to work out. So let Janie know if you discover one.

How do I treat excess RT3?

Patients have had success with three strategies:

Lower your NDT! For years, we thought that the only way to lower high RT3 was to be on T3-only. But we then discovered that one can simply move down on their NDT and accomplish the same thing, such as 1 1/2 grains or less. Some then add in some T3. It can take anywhere from 8 – 12 weeks to fully lower high RT3. If one was on synthetic T4 with synthetic T3 with high RT3, patients tend to scrap the T4 totally and just use the T3.

Identifying the causes and treating them: After either lowering our NDT or being on T3-only, we then treat the causes. You can read about iron, or cortisol, and how we treat them. See the Odds and Ends chapter in the revised STTM book for more about iron, and Chapter 6 on the use of HC or Adrenal Cortex. Also, changing your lifestyle can be key, as well, such as greatly improving your food choices, facing an alcohol addiction, stop smoking, and avoiding high stress.

Using a good liver cleanse/support product, plus Selenium: Since the bulk of RT3 is made in the liver, some have lowered their high RT3 by using a good liver cleanse, especially those with Milk Thistle. You may have to DOUBLE the recommended amount to get the lowered RT3. Milk Thistle can supposedly lower ferritin, so patients are adding iron to their supplementation, or raising what they are already on. Also make sure your Milk Thistle comes from the seeds. Milk Thistle not from the seeds can have an estrogenic effect. Also, there is a lot of research which proves that low selenium can increase RT3. So patients supplement with Selenium to stop that fact."

Her Hair Was Scraggly…(continued)

She came in the Green Room and sat down. She looked stressed and haggard.

"What happened?"

"I felt marvelous and then went back to my family doctor. He said my TSH was suppressed and I was on too much thyroid. That it would give me osteoporosis."

"That's an old doctor's tale. It won't. And your TSH was suppressed and worthless anyway."

"Then he looked though my labs and told me I didn't have hypothyroidism. That I should stop everything."

"How long ago did you stop it all?"

"Four months."

I looked at her directly and smiled. "So, what do you believe now – your own lying eyes? Or his doctor lips?"

She thought a second. "Well, I'm back here. So I think I believe my own lying eyes. I never felt so good than when I was on all that. And I feel horrible now – and my hair's falling out again."

"So what do you want to do?"

"Go back on it – on everything – can I or do we need to do all the testing again?"

"No. That's senseless – you can just start where you were. What about your family doc? What will he say?"

"What family doc? Who?"

My smile was grim. He could have called me and should have. I'm his Utah Medical Association County rep and was easy to get in contact. I let it go.

"Do you know a good primary care physician who can read labs and knows what you do?

I nodded. "I know several – some of them are patients (I can't tell you which though). Just never stop your thyroid again. Listen to your heart. Listen to your body."

She nodded. I noticed she was crying a little. She wiped a tear.

I started writing prescriptions.

CHAPTER 11

SIDE EFFECTS & PROBLEMS

Possible Side Effects of Too Much Thyroid (Exogenous Hyperthyroidism)

Insomnia.

Feeling hot or hot flashes.

Anxiety.

Nervousness.

Hypocholesterolemia[108]

Right Ventricular Hypertrophy, atrial fibrillation (4.00%), ventricular premature beats (2.77%), paroxysmal supraventricular tachycardia (2.23%), atrial flutter (1.00%).

Congestive heart failure occurred in 10.42% of the cases in one review[109].

Dementia (long-term extreme hyperthyroidism according to the Rotterdam Study)[110].

Refractory SVT[111] (supraventricular tachycardia).

One last thought...

REMINDER: Please leave a review if you enjoyed this book.

Thanks!

If this book has helped you in any way – brought some clarity to this problem in your life or answered some questions you had -- it might help someone else too. I'm certainly not asking a ton for this book but THE best way to pay it forward is by writing a review of this book to let others know of the benefits you've got from it. This will not only help others reach their health goals, but it is incredibly rewarding for me to know how much this work has benefited others, as well as learning any ways I can improve.... This way you can help empower others in the way this [book] has empowered you.

—*Dan*

Purser MD

Want to Connect with Dr. Purser?

MEN: To download THREE FREE REPORTS full of helpful **MEN**'s information on testosterone issues and other medical problems and as a BONUS my DR PURSER LAB SOUTIONS REPORT just clink on the link here:
http://www.drpursergift.com

For Dr. Purser's Amazon Author Page linking to all of his books (including his five #1 books):
http://www.greatmedebooks.com

To get to know Dr. Purser better and to get his email newsletter (full of discounts and coupons and freebies): http://drpurser.com

WOMEN: For **WOMEN**'s information on their health issues (PMS, migraines, endometriosis, menopause, thyroid, and osteoporosis)
http://www.drpursergift4women.com

Facebook: Dan Purser MD

Twitter #danpursermd

Pinterest: Dan Purser MD

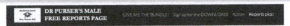

DR PURSER'S MALE FREE REPORTS PAGE — GIVE ME THE BUNDLE! · Sign up for the DOWNLOAD! · Action · Reports pics!

The REPORTS You Get!

YOU NEED THESE -- PLUS YOUR BONUS LAB REPORT!

Low levels of testosterone can be treated naturally & optimally in the right situations.	Questions I hear all the time from men regarding their low libido & testosterone. YOU SHOULD ASK THESE!	An AMAZING LIST every man should own -- all REFERENCED! NO FOOLING.	Detailed info on Lab Levels & Where to Get them CHEAP when your doc won't!

Sign up TODAY to Get Your FREE Reports!

Add text here.

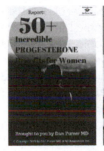 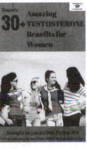 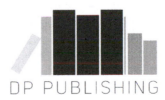

Add text here. · Add text here. · Add text here.

Low levels of progesterone can be treated naturally & optimally in the right situations.	An AMAZING LIST every woman should own -- all REFERENCED! NO FOOLING.	Detailed info on Lab Levels & Where to Get them CHEAP when your doc won't!

© Copyright by Dan Purser MD of DP Publishing

DP PUBLISHING

Index

A

Acne, 46
Activity, 21
  thyroid receptor, 21
Adaptogen, 54
Adrenal glands, 64
Adrenals, 64
Aging, 19, 20, 26, 63,
Alopecia, 34, 50
Amounts, 26, 38, 56, 64
  healthy, 65
  high, 64
  physiological, 21
  producing excessive, 64
  trace, 45
Androgenic hair loss, 13
Angina, 11, 24, 38, 41
Antibodies, 56–57, 59
  abnormal, 56
  autoimmune, 62
Antibody test, 56
Armour, 10, 14, 17, 19, 21, 22, 23, 24, 40
  benefit, 20
Atherosclerosis, 75
Attention Deficit Disorders, 46

B

Batch, 23
Berries, 53, 54
Beta conversion method, 66
Beware, 30, 48, 50
Bianchi, 78
Blood, 8, 17, 36, 64
Blood brain barrier, 27, 51
Blood-brain-barrier, 42
Blood tests, 56
  mineral panel, 16
Body, 19, 47, 63, 64, 69

Body's activities, 58
Body temperature, normal, 20
Brain fatigue, 42
Brain fog, 42, 51
Bromide overload, 45
Bromides, 45, 46
Bromine, 44, 45–46

C

Cardiac output, 12, 27, 28
Cells, red blood, 64
CHF, 12, 43
Children, 46, 47, 58
Chinese patients, 49
Cholesterol, total, 12
Chronic fatigue patients, 28
Chronic stresses, 63–64
Clinical symptom index, 12
Clinical symptoms, 37
Coal, selenium-rich stony, 49
Company Allegedly Hid Thyroid Research, 22
Concentration, 76
  highest, 49
Concurrent symptoms, 37
Constipation, 4, 8, 11
Contributor, 45
Conversion, 19, 63, 64
Convoluted twisted reasoning, 15
CoQ10, 27, 43
Cortisol, 64, 67
  excess, 64
  high, 63–64
  low, 64
Cortisol problem, 65
Critical Point, 37–38

D

Deficiencies, 33, 36, 48, 50
  intracellular, 33

vitamin, 33
Deiodination receptors, 19
Depression, 13, 20, 28, 29
Depression symptoms,
    improved, 28
Desiccated thyroid, 21, 24,
    28, 38, 39, 41
Diabetes, 19, 21, 63
Diagnosis, 11, 25, 56
Diet, 46, 49
DirectLabs, 66
Disorders
    autoimmune, 56
    gastrointestinal, 49
    genetics, 20
    neurodevelopmental, 46
    thyroid-resistant, 29
Doctors, 4, 8, 11, 15, 24,
    25, 34, 43, 57, 66, 68
Dose, 13, 28, 38, 40, 41,
    46, 49, 52, 60
    correct, 48
    daily, 40
    good, 48
    higher, 30
    low, 28
    massive, 27
    smallest, 30

E

Effect thyroid production,
    33
Elemental selenium, 49
Elevation, 11, 13
Engines, 34
Enzyme, deiodinase, 29, 48
Essential Oils, 6, 53, 82
Essential oil work, 54

F

Fatigue, 4, 8, 11, 12, 20,
    30, 37, 49
    adrenal, 64

Fatigue wall, 43
Federal Register, 22, 24, 25
Fibromyalgia, 13, 29
Flour, 44, 45
Foods, 24, 44, 45, 46
    natural, 47
France for normalizing
    hormonal imbalances,
    54
Free T3, 14, 28, 37, 38, 39,
    51, 60, 65, 66
Free T3 levels, 10, 11, 37–
    39
Free T4, 14, 26, 28, 38, 42,
    51, 59, 60, 65
FT3, 30, 33, 65
Functionality, 48, 50
Functions, 19, 34

G

Generations, 4
Girelli, 80, 81
Gland, 48, 50, 54–55, 58
    overactive, 54
Grain BID, 28
Grain of Armour, 40
Grain of NatureThroid, 40
Grains, 11, 13, 14, 17, 27,
    38, 39, 40, 52, 66
Grave's Disease, 6, 62
Great Hormone, 6

H

Hair, 7, 14, 31, 51, 60, 68
Hair dyes, 45
Hair loss, 7, 8, 30, 34, 49,
    50
    diffuse, 13
Hair regrowth, good, 13
Hashimoto's disease, 56,
    58
Hashimoto's Thyroiditis, 6,
    56, 58

Hashomoto's Thyroiditis, 62
hGH, 21
Higher dose treatment, 28
High RT3, 65, 66, 67
  lower, 66
Home page, 66
Hormones, 10, 25, 27, 29,
    56, 58, 63
  active, 38, 63
  active thyroid, 10, 20
  deiodinated thyroid, 21
  desiccated bovine, 23
  free T3, 29
  lesser-understood
    deiodinated thyroid, 21
  resistance to thyroid, 30,
    41
  storage, 63
Hormone test, 56
Human body, 20, 54
Hypercholesterolemia, 29
  iodine-induced, 44
  long-term extreme, 70
Hypothyroid, 14, 15, 30, 48,
    50
Hypothyroidism, 11, 12, 13,
    19, 20, 29, 37, 38, 58,
    75, 76
  overt, 48, 76
  tissue, 66

I

Increased hair and nail
    thickness, 26
Increased immune
    resistance, 26
Inflammation, 53, 58
Intracellular vitamin, 16
Intracellular vitamin panels,
    50
Iodide, 45, 47–48
Iodide capsule, 48
Iodide transporters, 47

Iodine, 43, 44, 45, 46, 47,
    48
  bound, 46
  natural, 45
  supersaturated, 47
  transports, 47
Iodine capsules, 43, 48
  best, 48
Iodine deficiency, 44, 45
Iodine Deficiency Disorder,
    44, 48
Iodine deficit, 45
Iodine levels, 45, 46
Iodine receptors, 45
Iodine's disappearance, 44
Iodine supplements, 44
Ionized form, 47
Iron, 64, 67
Iron levels, 64
Iron problems, 65

J

Jaw, 15

L

Labs, 14, 15, 25, 30, 37,
    68, 69
Labwork, 66
Levothyroxine, 24, 75, 81
Levo-thyroxine, 38, 42
Levothyroxine, synthetic, 25
Levo-thyroxine therapy, 76
Liothyronine, 28, 75
Literature receptor
    problems, 14
Liver, 49, 53, 63, 67
Liver cleanse, good, 67
Low-Dose, 75
Low T3, 38
Low TSH, 39, 41
l-thyroxine, 22, 76
L-Thyroxine, 75
l-thyroxine

excess, 24
little, 4

M

Manufacture, 48, 50
Marchesini, 78
Mayo Clinic, 56, 58
Medical Crossfire, 75
Medscape, 77
Metabolism, 75
Metallic selenides, 49
Middle-aged women, 58
Migraines, 73
Milk Thistle, 67
Molecule, 47
Morkin, 78
Muscle cramps, 11, 16
Myrtle, 53, 54
  common, 53
  creeping, 54
  crepe, 54
  wax, 54
Myrtle berries, 54
Myrtle oil, 54
  researched, 54
Myrtle Oil Normalizes, 54
Myrtus communis, 53, 54
Myth, 25

N

Nature-Throid, 16–17, 51
NDT, 66–67
Normalizing hormonal
    imbalances, 54
Normal ranges, 25
Nuclear receptor mRNA
    expression, 77
Nuclear retinoid receptors
    for thyroid, 19
Nutrients, 47, 49

O

Oil, 54
Old physician's wives tales,
    4
Olivieri, 80, 81
Osteoporosis, 13, 68, 73
Outlawed bromide, 46
Ovaries, 54
Overt symptoms, 29
Oxidative stress, 47

P

Patients, 3, 10, 12, 26, 28,
    30, 37, 38–41, 43, 57,
    65, 66, 76
  high-end, 8
  hypothyroid, 12, 38
  rare, 27
Patients benefit, 10
Patients supplement, 67
Patient's symptoms stem,
    37
Peer Exchange, 80
Peripheral receptor sites,
    27
Peripheral tissues, 21, 30,
    37
Personal Beliefs on Thyroid
    Dosing, 11
Physician monitoring, 11
Physicians, 4, 21, 22, 25,
    28
  good primary care, 69
  knowledgeable, 3
Pituitary, 15, 25, 26
  suppressed, 26
Pituitary glands, 56
Plugs, 34
Pool, 64
Porcine thyroid, 23
  desiccated, 21, 23, 25
Post-menopausal women,
    13, 76

Potassium bromate, 45
Potency, 23
  consistent, 22, 24
Primary Hypothyroidism, 75
Products, 40, 45, 46
  administered
    levothyroxine sodium,
    22, 24
Pseudo-hypothyroidism, 50
Purser's Amazon Author
  Page linking, 73

R

Radioactive iodine, 45
Range, 53, 54, 65
Rasgon, 78, 79
Ratio, 65, 66
  rT3, 66
Ratio comparison, 66
Rationalize, 13
Ratio result, 65
Reason, 13, 21, 57, 63
  sheer, 19
Receptor exhaustion, 19
Receptor failure, 13, 37, 38
  insulin, 20–21
  thyroid T3, 37
Receptors, 21, 27, 33, 34,
  50
  faulty, 41
  peripheral retinoid, 19
  peripheral T3, 27
Recurrent Pregnancy Loss,
  79
Resistance, 19, 30, 41, 76
  insulin, 21, 34
  organ, 21
Reverse T3, 6, 63, 65
Rough Conversion
    Formula, 14
RT3, 63, 64, 65, 67
  excess, 64, 66

S

Seeds, 67
Selenium, 29, 48–50, 62,
  67
  element, 29
  ingested, 49
  low, 67
Selenium Capsules, 48
Selenium content, 49
Selenium deficiency, 33
Selenium supplementation
  in thyroid, 83
Selenium toxicity, 49
Selenosis, 49
Serum Lipids, 75
SINGLE ESSENTIAL OILS
    Myrtle Essential Oil,
    53
Skin, dry, 4, 11, 20
Slenites, 50
Slid, 8, 14, 17
Slow-Release
    Triiodothyronine
    Replacement in
    Hypothyroidism, 75
Sodium-iodide symporter,
  47
Spectracell, 31, 36, 60
Stability, 22, 24
Stew, healthy, 24
Stomach, empty, 11
Stop, 16, 52, 67, 68, 69
Storage hormone T4, 63
Subclinical hypothyroidism,
  11–13, 28, 29, 75, 76,
  77, 79–80
Subclinical hypothyroid
  women, 13
Subjects, 11–12
  healthy, 80, 81
Supplement, 47, 48
  good zinc, 50
Supplementation, 11, 67

Supplementing, 12
Support Thyroid Function,
    6, 53
Suppress, 11, 25, 27, 59
Supraphysiologic doses,
    13, 29
Symptom, right, 15
Symptoms, 11, 13, 20, 24,
    29, 37, 41, 49, 56, 64
Synthetic T3, 21, 25, 66
Synthroid, 10, 14, 16, 21,
    22–23
System
  cardiovascular, 78, 79
  human thyroid, 19
  porcine thyroid, 19

T

Thyroglobulin, 47
Thyroid, 6, 8, 10, 12, 13,
    15, 19, 21, 25–28, 41,
    47, 54, 56
  desiccated animal, 10, 25
  dessicated, 23
  endogenous, 27
  extra, 26
  healthy, 63
  human, 23
  low, 16
  sustained release, 40
  weird animal, 24
Thyroid activity, 54
Thyroid Agents, 75
Thyroid care, 37
Thyroid condition, 47
Thyroid Dosing, 11
Thyroid dysfunction, 48, 75,
    76
Thyroid-energy pathways,
    26
Thyroid experts, 11
Thyroid failure, 29
  moderate, 29
  total, 29

Thyroid function, 6, 43, 58,
    77, 82
Thyroid gland, 25, 47, 56–
    58
  underactive, 58
Thyroid health, 54
Thyroid hormone, 12, 19,
    25–30, 34, 38, 41, 42,
    44, 48, 50, 56–57, 64,
    76
Thyroid hormone
    deiodinases, 82
Thyroid Hormone
    Generating System,
    77
Thyroid hormone
    replacement, 58
Thyroid Hormone
    Replacement Therapy
    in Primary
    Hypothyroidism, 75
Thyroid hormone
    resistance, 13, 20, 76,
    77
Thyroid hormone
    supplementation, 10
Thyroid illness, 25
Thyroid inadequacy, 39
Thyroid issues, 3
Thyroiditis, chronic
    lymphocytic, 58
Thyroid levels, 35, 39, 43
Thyroid Manager, 78
Thyroid patients, 63–64
Thyroid peroxidase, 56
Thyroid Practice Gems, 6,
    40
Thyroid problems, 3, 4, 37
Thyroid production, 19
Thyroid profile, 51
Thyroid receptor failure, 20
Thyroid receptors, 19, 20,
    34
Thyroid receptor site, 48,
    50

Thyroid reserve, 76
Thyroid resistance, 14, 19,
    20, 30, 33, 34
Thyroid resistance cases,
    21
Thyroid sensitivity, 38
Thyroid-stimulating
    hormone
    . See TSH
    normal, 38
Thyroid supplementation,
    26, 28
Thyroid tissue levels, 65
Thyrotropin, 76
Thyroxine, 75, 76
Thyroxine replacement, 13
Time, 4, 7, 13, 33, 43, 56,
    66
Tolerable Upper Intake
    Level, 49
TPO antibodies, 15
Treatment, 3, 25, 29, 40,
    53, 57, 58, 75
    inadequate, 64
Treatment option, cheap,
    13
Treatment protocol, 44
Triiodothyronine, 75, 76
    intravenous, 76
TSH (thyroid-stimulating
    hormone), 8, 11, 14,
    25, 28, 29, 37, 38–39,
    56, 59, 68
TSH levels, 10, 11, 26, 27,
    37, 39, 41
TSH range, 25

U

Unrelated plants, 54
Use L-thyroxine, 10

V

Vascular resistance, 12
    increased, 27
    systemic, 27
Vitamins, 6, 16, 35–36, 43,
    60

W

Warmer body temperature,
    26
Water, 44–45
Weight, 15, 20, 27
    kilogram body, 49
Weight loss, 12, 26, 41
WHO (World Health
    Organization), 44, 45
Women, 4, 13, 27, 43, 50,
    58, 73, 75
World Health Organization
    (WHO), 44, 45

Z

Zalinkevicius, 75, 76, 79
Zinc, 16, 27, 50
Zinc deficiency, 27, 34, 50
Zinc Tablets, 50

REFERENCES

[1] No author listed. Available at http://www.drugs.com/drug-class/thyroid-drugs.html. Accessed 16 April 2015.

[2] Bunevicius R, Kazanavicius G, Zalinkevicius R, Prange AJ Jr. Effects of thyroxine as compared with thyroxine plus triiodothyronine in patients with hypothyroidism. N Engl J Med. 1999 Feb 11;340(6):424-9.

[3] Escobar-Morreale, H. F., Botella-Carretero, J. I., del Rey, F. E., de Escobar, G. M. (2005). Treatment of Hypothyroidism with Combinations of Levothyroxine plus Liothyronine. *J Clin Endocrinol Metab* 90: 4946-4954

[4] Escobar-Morreale, H. F., Botella-Carretero, J. I., Gomez-Bueno, M., Galan, J. M., Barrios, V., Sancho, J. (2005). Thyroid Hormone Replacement Therapy in Primary Hypothyroidism: A Randomized Trial Comparing L-Thyroxine plus Liothyronine with L-Thyroxine Alone. *Ann Intern Med* 142: 412-424

[5] Hennemann, G. Thyroxine Plus Low-Dose, Slow-Release Triiodothyronine Replacement in Hypothyroidism: Proof of Principle. Thyroid. Apr 2004, Vol. 14, No. 4: 271 -275.

[6] www.synthroidclaims.com

[7] Beckett GJ, Toft AD First-line thyroid function tests-TSH alone is not enough
Clin Endocrinol 2003; 56; 20-1.

[8] Arafah B. M. Increased Need for Thyroxine in Women with Hypothyroidism during Estrogen Therapy. N Engl J Med 2001; 344:1743-1749, Jun 7, 2001.

[9] AHFS Drug Information.(68:36.04 Thyroid Agents.) AHFS Drug Information (2004). Via Stat!Ref online. Available at: http://online.statref.com/. Accessed on November 23, 2004.

[10] [no author listed] What is Subclinical Hypothyroidism? Medical Crossfire. December 2000; Vol 2, No 12.

[11] Walsh, JP; Bremner,AP; Bulsara, MK; O'Leary, P; Leedman, PJ; Feddema, P; Michelangeli, V. Thyroid Dysfunction and Serum Lipids: A Community-Based Study. Clin Endocrinol. 2005;63(3):670-675. ©2005 Blackwell Publishing.

[12] Walsh, JP; Bremner,AP; Bulsara, MK; O'Leary, P; Leedman, PJ; Feddema, P; Michelangeli, V. Thyroid Dysfunction and Serum Lipids: A Community-Based Study. Clin Endocrinol. 2005;63(3):670-675. ©2005 Blackwell Publishing.

[13] Cappola, A.R. & Ladenson, P.W. (2003) Hypothyroidism and atherosclerosis. Journal of Clinical Endocrinology and Metabolism, 88, 2438– 2444.

[14] Cappola, A.R. & Ladenson, P.W. (2003) Hypothyroidism and atherosclerosis. Journal of Clinical Endocrinology and Metabolism, 88, 2438– 2444.

[15] Landenson PW. Recognition and management of cardiovascular disease related to thyroid dysfunction. Am J Med 1990;88:638-41.

[16] Hamilton MA, Stevenson LW, Fonarow GC, Steimle A, Goldhaber JI, Child JS, Chopra IJ, Moriguchi JD, Hage A. Safety and hemodynamic effects of intravenous triiodothyronine in advanced congestive heart failure. Am J Cardiol. 1998 Feb 15;81(4):443-7.

[17] P. Saravanan, W.-F. Chau, N. Roberts, K. Vedhara, R. Greenwood and C. M. Dayan. (2002) Psychological well-being in patients on 'adequate' doses of l-thyroxine: results of a large, controlled community-based questionnaire study. *Clinical Endocrinology* **57**:5, 577-585

[18] Cooper, DS. Subclinical Thyroid Disease: A Clinician's Perspective. Annals of Internal Medicine. 15 July 1998; Volume 129: Issue 2: Pages 135-138

[19] Surks MI, Ocampo E. Subclinical thyroid disease. Am J Med. 1996; 100:217-23

[20] Staub JJ, Althaus BU, Engler H, Ryff AS, Trabucco P, Marquardt K, et al. Spectrum of subclinical and overt hypothyroidism: effect on thyrotropin, prolactin, and thyroid reserve, and metabolic impact on peripheral target tissues. Am J Med. 1992; 92:631-41.

[21] Yildirimkaya M, Ozata M, Yilmaz K, Kilinc C, Gundogan MA, Kutluay T. Lipoprotein(a) concentration in subclinical hypothyroidism before and after levo-thyroxine therapy. Endocr J. 1996; 43:731-6.

[22] Bunevicius R, Kazanavicius G, Zalinkevicius R, Prange AJ Jr. Effects of thyroxine as compared with thyroxine plus triiodothyronine in patients with hypothyroidism. N Engl J Med. 1999 Feb 11;340(6):469-70.

[23] Barbara Baker "No BMD Loss With Thyroid Replacement Tx". OB/GYN News. Sept 1, 2000. FindArticles.com. 09 Oct. 2006.

[24] Kuijpens JL, Nyklictek I, Louwman MW, Weetman TA, Pop VJ, Coebergh JW. Hypothyroidism might be related to breast cancer in post-menopausal women. Thyroid. 2005 Nov;15(11):1253-9.

[25] Garrison RL, Breeding PC. A metabolic basis for fibromyalgia and its related disorders: the possible role of resistance to thyroid hormone. Med Hypotheses. 2003 Aug;61(2):182-9.

[26] Beck-Peccoz P, Mannavola D, Persani L. Syndromes of thyroid hormone resistance. Ann Endocrinol (Paris). 2005 Jun;66(3):264-9.

[27] Tjorve E, Tjorve KM, Olsen JO, Senum R, Oftebro H. On commonness and rarity of thyroid hormone resistance: A discussion based on mechanisms of reduced sensitivity in peripheral tissues. Med Hypotheses. 2007 Mar 23.

[28] [no author listed] What is Subclinical Hypothyroidism? Medical Crossfire. December 2000; Vol 2, No 12.

[29] Feart C, Pallet V, Boucheron C, Higueret D, Alfos S, Letenneur L, Dartigues JF, Higueret P. Aging affects the retinoic acid and the triiodothyronine nuclear receptor mRNA expression in human peripheral blood mononuclear cells. Eur J Endocrinol. 2005 Mar;152(3):449-58.

[30] Takashi Akamizu, Leonard D. Kohn, Hitomi Hiratani, Misa Saijo, Kazuo Tahara and Kazuwa Nakao. Special Articles: Hashimoto's Thyroiditis with Heterogeneous Antithyrotropin Receptor Antibodies: Unique Epitopes May Contribute to the Regulation of Thyroid Function by the Antibodies1. The Journal of Clinical Endocrinology & Metabolism Vol. 85, No. 6 2116-2121. Copyright © 2000 by The Endocrine Society.

[31] Brucker-Davis F, Skarulis MC, Grace MB, Benichou J, Hauser P, Wiggs E, et al. Genetic and clinical features of 42 kindreds with resistance to thyroid hormone. The National Institutes of Health Prospective Study. Ann Intern Med. 1995; 123:572-83.

[32] Durrant-Peatfield B. Thyroid and adrenal dysfunction: the diagnosis and treatment of an endemic syndrome. Institute for Complementary Medicine, February 2006 Edition.

[33] Noth RH, Mazzaferri EL. Age and the endocrine system. Clin Geriatr Med. 1985 Feb;1(1):223-50.

[34] Knobel M, Medeiros-Neto G. An Outline of Inherited Disorders of the Thyroid Hormone Generating System. Thyroid 13(8):771-801, 2003. © 2003 Mary Ann Liebert, Inc.

[35] Burman, KD. Clinical Management of Hypothyroidism. [online] Available on Medscape® at /www.medscape.com/viewprogram/706. Accessed 2006 Sep 8.

[36] Burman, KD. Clinical Management of Hypothyroidism. [online] Available on Medscape at /www.medscape.com/viewprogram/706. Accessed 2006 Sep 8.

[37] Ghafoor F, Mansoor M, Malik T, Malik MS, Khan AU, Edwards R, Akhtar W. Role of thyroid peroxidase antibodies in

the outcome of pregnancy. J Coll Physicians Surg Pak. 2006 Jul;16(7):468-71.

[38] Burman, KD. Clinical Management of Hypothyroidism: Thyroid Hormone Resistance. [online] Available on Medscape® at /www.medscape.com/viewprogram/706. Accessed 2006 Sep 9.

[39] Chatterjee VK. Resistance to thyroid hormone, and peroxisome-proliferator-activated receptor gamma resistance. Biochem Soc Trans. 2001; 29(Pt 2):227-31 (ISSN: 0300-5127).

[40] Rezvani I., DiGeorge AM, Dowshen SA, Bourdony CJ. Action of human growth hormone (hGH) on extrathyroidal conversion of thyroxine (T4) to triiodothyronine (T3) in children with hypopituitarism. Pediatric Research, Vol 15, 6-9, Copyright © 1981 by International Pediatric Research Foundation.

[41] De Groot, Leslie J. M.D., Georg Hennemann, M.D., Thyroid Manager, December 2002. http://www.thyroidmanager.org/Chapter6/Ch-6-3.htm.

[42] Fazio S, Palmieri EA, Lombardi G, Biondi B. Effects of thyroid hormone on the cardiovascular system. Recent Prog Horm Res. 2004;59:31-50.

[43] De Groot, Leslie J. M.D., Georg Hennemann, M.D., Thyroid Manager, December 2002. http://www.thyroidmanager.org/Chapter6/Ch-6-3.htm

[44] Bianchi G, Solaroli E, Zaccheroni V, Grossi G, Bargossi AM, Melchionda N, Marchesini G. Oxidative stress and anti-oxidant metabolites in patients with hyperthyroidism: effect of treatment. Horm Metab Res. 1999 Nov;31(11):620-4.

[45] Morkin E; Ladenson P; Goldman S; Adamson C. Thyroid hormone analogs for treatment of hypercholesterolemia and heart failure: past, present and future prospects. J Mol Cell Cardiol. 2004; 37(6):1137-46 (ISSN: 0022-2828).

[46] Morkin E; Ladenson P; Goldman S; Adamson C. Thyroid hormone analogs for treatment of hypercholesterolemia and heart failure: past, present and future prospects. J Mol Cell Cardiol. 2004; 37(6):1137-46 (ISSN: 0022-2828).

[47] Danzi S, Klein I. Thyroid hormone and the cardiovascular system. Minerva Endocrinol. 2004 Sep;29(3):139-50.

[48] Barbara Baker "No BMD Loss With Thyroid Replacement Tx". OB/GYN News. Sept 1, 2000. FindArticles.com. 09 Oct. 2006.

[49] Wartofsky L, Van Nostrand D, Burman KD. Overt and 'subclinical' hypothyroidism in women. Obstet Gynecol Surv. 2006 Aug;61(8):535-42.

[50] Miller KJ, Parsons TD, Whybrow PC, van Herle K, Rasgon N, van Herle A, Martinez D, Silverman DH, Bauer M. Memory improvement with treatment of hypothyroidism. Int J Neurosci. 2006 Aug;116(8):895-906.

[51] Friesema EC, Jansen J, Visser TJ. Thyroid hormone transporters. Biochem Soc Trans. 2005 Feb;33(Pt 1):228-32.

[52] Bianchi G, Solaroli E, Zaccheroni V, Grossi G, Bargossi AM, Melchionda N, Marchesini G. Oxidative stress and anti-oxidant metabolites in patients with hyperthyroidism: effect of treatment. Horm Metab Res. 1999 Nov;31(11):620-4.

[53] Freake HC; Govoni KE; Guda K; Huang C; Zinn SA. Actions and interactions of thyroid hormone and zinc status in growing rats. J Nutr. 2001; 131(4):1135-41 (ISSN: 0022-3166).

[54] Danzi S; Klein I. Thyroid hormone and the cardiovascular system. Minerva Endocrinol. 2004; 29(3):139-50 (ISSN: 0391-1977).

[55] Danzi S, Klein I. Thyroid hormone and the cardiovascular system. Minerva Endocrinol. 2004 Sep;29(3):139-50.

[56] Kovacs, P. Recurrent Pregnancy Loss. [online] Available at www.medscape.com/viewprogram/5293_pnt. Accessed 2006 Oct 13. Copyright © 2006 Medscape.

[57] Ables AZ, Baughman OL 3rd. Antidepressants: update on new agents and indications. Am Fam Physician. 2003 Feb 1;67(3):547-54.

[58] Bunevicius R, Kazanavicius G, Zalinkevicius R, Prange AJ Jr. Effects of thyroxine as compared with thyroxine plus triiodothyronine in patients with hypothyroidism. N Engl J Med. 1999 Feb 11;340(6):424-9.

[59] McGrath PJ, Quitkin FM, Klein DF. Bromocriptine treatment of relapses seen during selective serotonin re-uptake inhibitor treatment of depression [letter]. J Clin Psychopharmacol. 1995;15:289-291.

[60] Pallotti S, Gasbarrone A, Franzese IT. [Relationship between insulin secretion, and thyroid and ovary function in patients suffering from polycystic ovary][Article in Italian] Minerva Endocrinol. 2005 Sep;30(3):193-7.

[61] Gerwin RD. A review of myofascial pain and fibromyalgia--factors that promote their persistence. Acupunct Med. 2005 Sep;23(3):121-34.

[62] Smallridge RC. Disclosing subclinical thyroid disease. An approach to mild laboratory abnormalities and vague or absent symptoms. Postgrad Med. 2000 Jan;107(1):143-6, 149-52.

[63] Miller KJ, Parsons TD, Whybrow PC, van Herle K, Rasgon N, van Herle A, Martinez D, Silverman DH, Bauer M. Memory improvement with treatment of hypothyroidism. Int J Neurosci. 2006 Aug;116(8):895-906.

[64] Oerbeck B, Sundet K, Kase BF, Heyerdahl S. Congenital hypothyroidism: no adverse effects of high dose thyroxine treatment on adult memory, attention, and behaviour. Arch Dis Child. 2005 Feb;90(2):132-7.

[65] Garrison RL, Breeding PC. A metabolic basis for fibromyalgia and its related disorders: the possible role of resistance to thyroid hormone. Med Hypotheses. 2003 Aug;61(2):182-9.

[66] Tseng FY, Lin WY, et al. Subclinical hypothyroidism is associated with increased risk for cancer mortality in adult taiwanese-a 10 years population-based cohort. PLoS One. 2015 Apr 1;10(4):e0122955. doi: 10.1371/journal.pone.0122955. eCollection 201

[67] Rubin, AL. Subclinical Hypothyroidism. Medical Crossfire, Peer Exchange. December 2000. Available online at /www.medicalcrossfire.com.

[68] Bunevicius R, Jakubonien N, Jurkevicius R, Cernicat J, Lasas L, Prange AJ Jr. Thyroxine vs thyroxine plus triiodothyronine in treatment of hypothyroidism after thyroidectomy for Graves' disease. Endocrine. 2002 Jul;18(2):129-33.

[69] [no author listed] [online] Available at www.clinicaltrials.gov/ct/show/NCT00106119. Accessed 2006 Oct 13.

[70] Jaffiol C, Baldet L, Torresani J, Bismuth J, Papachristou C. A case of hypersensitivity to thyroid hormones with normally functioning thyroid gland and increased nuclear triiodothyronine receptors. J Endocrinol Invest. 1990 Nov;13(10):839-45. Jaffiol C, Baldet L, Torresani J, Bismuth J, Papachristou C. A case of hypersensitivity to thyroid hormones with normally functioning thyroid gland and increased nuclear triiodothyronine receptors. J Endocrinol Invest. 1990 Nov;13(10):839-45.

[71] Rubin, AL. Subclinical Hypothyroidism. Medical Crossfire, Peer Exchange. December 2000. Available online at /www.medicalcrossfire.com.

[72] Weiss, RE, Dumitrescu, A, et al. Approach to the Patient with Resistance to Thyroid Hormone and Pregnancy. J Clin Endocrinol Metab. 2010 July; 95(7): 3094–3102. doi: 10.1210/jc.2010-0409.

[73] Chantler, D, Moran, C, et al. Resistance to thyroid hormone – an incidental finding. BMJ Case Rep. 2012; 2012: bcr1220115375.

[74] Alevizaki M, Mantzou E, Cimponeriu AT, Alevizaki CC, Koutras DA. TSH may not be a good marker for adequate thyroid hormone replacement therapy. Wien Klin Wochenschr. 2005 Sep;117(18):636-40.

[75] Danzi S, Klein I. Potential uses of T3 in the treatment of human disease. Clin Cornerstone. 2005;7 Suppl 2:S9-15.

[76] Danzi S, Klein I. Potential uses of T3 in the treatment of human disease. Clin Cornerstone. 2005;7 Suppl 2:S9-15.

[77] Brucker-Davis F, Skarulis MC, Grace MB, Benichou J, Hauser P, Wiggs E, et al. Genetic and clinical features of 42 kindreds with resistance to thyroid hormone. The National Institutes of Health Prospective Study. Ann Intern Med. 1995; 123:572-83.

[78] Olivieri O, Girelli D, Stanzial AM, Rossi L, Bassi A, Corrocher R. Selenium, zinc, and thyroid hormones in healthy subjects: low T3/T4 ratio in the elderly is related to impaired selenium status. Biol Trace Elem Res. 1996 Jan;51(1):31-41.

[79] Santos GM, Pantoja CJ, Costa E Silva A, Rodrigues MC, Ribeiro RC, Simeoni LA, Lomri N, Neves FA. Thyroid hormone receptor binding to DNA and T3-dependent transcriptional activation are inhibited by uremic toxins.Nucl Recept. 2005 Apr 4;3(1):1.

[80] Oerbeck B, Sundet K, Kase BF, Heyerdahl S. Congenital hypothyroidism: no adverse effects of high dose thyroxine treatment on adult memory, attention, and behaviour. Arch Dis Child. 2005 Feb;90(2):132-7.

[81] Bunevicius R, Jakubonien N, Jurkevicius R, Cernicat J, Lasas L, Prange AJ Jr. Thyroxine vs thyroxine plus triiodothyronine in treatment of hypothyroidism after thyroidectomy for Graves' disease. Endocrine. 2002 Jul;18(2):129-33.

[82] Bindi M, Pinelli M, Rosada J, Castiglioni M. [Atrial fibrillation and thyroid gland][Article in Italian] Recenti Prog Med. 2005 Nov;96(11):548-51.

[83] Trivieri MG, Oudit GY, Sah R, Kerfant BG, Sun H, Gramolini AO, Pan Y, Wickenden AD, Croteau W, Morreale de Escobar G, Pekhletski R, St Germain D, Maclennan DH, Backx PH. Cardiac-specific elevations in thyroid hormone enhance contractility and prevent pressure overload-induced cardiac dysfunction. Proc Natl Acad Sci U S A. 2006 Apr 11;103(15):6043-8.

[84] Olivieri O, Girelli D, Stanzial AM, Rossi L, Bassi A, Corrocher R. Selenium, zinc, and thyroid hormones in healthy subjects: low T3/T4 ratio in the elderly is related to impaired selenium status. Biol Trace Elem Res. 1996 Jan;51(1):31-41.

[85] Brent GA. Mechanisms of thyroid hormone action. J Clin Invest. 2012;122(9):3035–3043.

[86] Fu A, Zhou R, et al. The synthetic thyroid hormone, levothyroxine, protects cholinergic neurons in the hippocampus of naturally aged mice. Neural Regen Res. 2014 Apr 15; 9(8): 864–871. doi: 10.4103/1673-5374.131602 PMCID: PMC4146262

[87] Mancini A, Corbo GM, et al. Relationships between plasma CoQ10 levels and thyroid hormones in chronic obstructive pulmonary disease. Biofactors. 2005;25(1-4):201-4.

[88] Littarru GP, Langsjoen P. Coenzyme Q10 and statins: biochemical and clinical implications. Mitochondrion. 2007 Jun;7 Suppl:S168-74. Epub 2007 Mar 27.

[89] Caldwell, K., et al. 2005; Hollowell, J., et al. 1998

[90] Pick, M NP. Accessed 19 May 2015 online at https://www.womentowomen.com/thyroid-health/iodine-and-the-thyroid-worth-a-second-glance/

[91] Mercola MD. Accessed 19 May 2015 online at http://articles.mercola.com/sites/articles/archive/2009/10/20/signs-symptoms-and-solutions-for-poor-thyroid-function.aspx

[92] Mercola MD. Accessed 19 May 2015 online at http://articles.mercola.com/sites/articles/archive/2009/10/20/signs-symptoms-and-solutions-for-poor-thyroid-function.aspx

[93] Mercola MD. Accessed 19 May 2015 online at http://articles.mercola.com/sites/articles/archive/2009/10/20/signs-symptoms-and-solutions-for-poor-thyroid-function.aspx

[94] Zimmermann MB, Bridson J, Bozo M, Grimci L, Selimaj V, Tanner MS. Severe iodine deficiency in southern Albania. Int J Vitam Nutr Res. 2003 Oct;73(5):347-50.

[95] Kvícala J, Zamrazil V. Effect of iodine and selenium upon thyroid function. Cent Eur J Public Health. 2003 Jun;11(2):107-13.

[96] Köhrle J. Thyroid hormone deiodinases--a selenoenzyme family acting as gate keepers to thyroid hormone action. Acta Med Austriaca. 1996;23(1-2):17-30.

[97] No author listed. Accessed 16 May 2015 online at http://www.news-medical.net/health/Selenium-Toxicity.aspx

[98] Freake HC, Govoni KE, et al. Actions and interactions of thyroid hormone and zinc status in growing rats. J Nutr. 2001 Apr;131(4):1135-41.

[99] Betsy A, Binitha M, Sarita S. Zinc deficiency associated with hypothyroidism: an overlooked cause of severe alopecia. Int J Trichology. 2013 Jan;5(1):40-2. doi: 10.4103/0974-7753.114714.

[100] Thomas, JP. Accessed 16 May 2015 online at http://healthimpactnews.com/2014/myrtle-essential-oil-normalizing-the-function-of-thyroid-and-ovaries/#sthash.lYdSfi22.dpuf

[101] "Review of Pharmacological Effects of Myrtus communis L. and its Active Constituents," Phytother Res. 2/4/2014, PMID: 24497171.

[102] The Chemistry of Essential Oils Made Simple – God's Love Manifest in Molecules, David Stewart, Ph.D., D.N.M., Integrated Aromatic Science Practitioner, Care Publications, Fourth Printing 2013, pp 60.

[103] The Chemistry of Essential Oils Made Simple – God's Love Manifest in Molecules, David Stewart, Ph.D., D.N.M., Integrated Aromatic Science Practitioner, Care Publications, Fourth Printing 2013, pp 248.

[104] Mayo Clinic Staff. Accessed 16 May 2015 online at http://www.mayoclinic.org/diseases-conditions/hashimotos-disease/basics/tests-diagnosis/con-20030293

[105] Mayo Clinic Staff. Accessed 16 May 2015 online at http://www.mayoclinic.org/diseases-conditions/hashimotos-disease/basics/definition/con-20030293

[106] No author listed. Accessed 05 November 2015 online at https://en.wikipedia.org/wiki/Graves%27_disease

[107] Dharmasena A. Selenium supplementation in thyroid associated ophthalmopathy: an update. Int J Ophthalmol. 2014 Apr 18;7(2):365-75. doi: 10.3980/j.issn.2222-3959.2014.02.31. eCollection 2014.

[108] Liberopoulos EN, Elisaf MS. Dyslipidemia in patients with thyroid disorders. Hormones (Athens). 2002 Oct-Dec;1(4):218-23.

[109] Vlase H, Lungu G, Vlase L. Cardiac disturbances in thyrotoxicosis: diagnosis, incidence, clinical features and management. Endocrinologie. 1991;29(3-4):155-60.

[110] Kalmijn S, Mehta KM, Pols HA, Hofman A, Drexhage HA, Breteler MM 2000 Subclinical hyperthyroidism and the risk of

dementia: The Rotterdam Study. Clin Endocrinol (Oxf) 53:733–737.

[111] Wald DA, Silver A. Cardiovascular manifestations of thyroid storm: a case report. J Emerg Med. 2003 Jul;25(1):23-8.

Made in the USA
Middletown, DE
09 January 2020

82886792R00056